Continuous Renal Replacement Therapy

Pittsburgh Critical Care Medicine

**Published and Forthcoming Books in
the Pittsburgh Critical Care Medicine series**

Continuous Renal Replacement Therapy

Second Edition

Edited by

John A. Kellum, MD, MCCM

Professor of Critical Care Medicine, Bioengineering and Clinical
    Translational Science
Director, Center for Critical Care Nephrology
Vice Chair for Research, Department of Critical Care Medicine
University of Pittsburgh School of Medicine
Pittsburgh, Pennsylvania

Rinaldo Bellomo, MBBS, MD, FRACP, FCICM

Director of Intensive Care Research
Department of Intensive Care
Austin Hospital
Victoria, Australia

Claudio Ronco, MD

Director, Department Nephrology Dialysis and Transplantation
Director of International Renal Research Institute (IRRIV)
San Bortolo Hospital
Vicenza, Italy

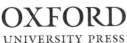

OXFORD
UNIVERSITY PRESS

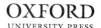

Library of Congress Cataloging-in-Publication Data
Continuous renal replacement therapy/edited by John A. Kellum, Rinaldo Bellomo,
and Claudio Ronco. — 2nd edition.
    p. ; cm.
Includes bibliographical references and index.
ISBN 978–0–19–022553–7 (alk. paper)
I. Kellum, John A., editor.   II. Bellomo, R. (Rinaldo), 1956– , editor.
III. Ronco, C. (Claudio), 1951– , editor.
[DNLM: 1. Acute Kidney Injury—therapy.   2. Hemodialysis Solutions.
3. Kidney—injuries.   4. Renal Replacement Therapy—methods.   WJ 342]
RC901.7.H45
617.4'61059—dc23
2015022091

9 8 7 6 5 4 3 2

Printed by Webcom, Canada

We dedicate this edition to the nursing professionals who deliver continuous renal replacement therapy. Without their hard work and dedication, this therapy would not exist. This volume is also dedicated to patients and their families in the hope that we make a positive difference in their lives.

Preface

Significant advances have occurred in the care of patients with acute kidney injury (AKI). Continuous renal replacement therapy (CRRT) has become standard of care for many critically ill patients with severe acute kidney injury, and most major medical centers have developed the capability of providing CRRT. However, many hospitals lack the capacity and many that have it, underuse it.

The goal of this CRRT handbook is to provide a concise but authoritative guide in the use of CRRT. In a single, slim volume, we cover the basics of CRRT management as well as some topics related more generally to AKI. The intent of this book is to provide a quick reference for both novice and experienced CRRT providers, to enrich existing expertise, and to help all involved in the care of severe AKI achieve a better understanding of this powerful therapy.

As a result of the tremendous success of the first edition, we have updated this second edition with new information on machines and biomarkers, and on a nomenclature that has undergone much-needed standardization during the years the first edition was published. We hope that new readers and those already familiar with the handbook find it useful. Our ultimate goal is to improve outcomes for patients with AKI through teamwork and education.

John A Kellum
Rinaldo Bellomo
Claudio Ronco
2015

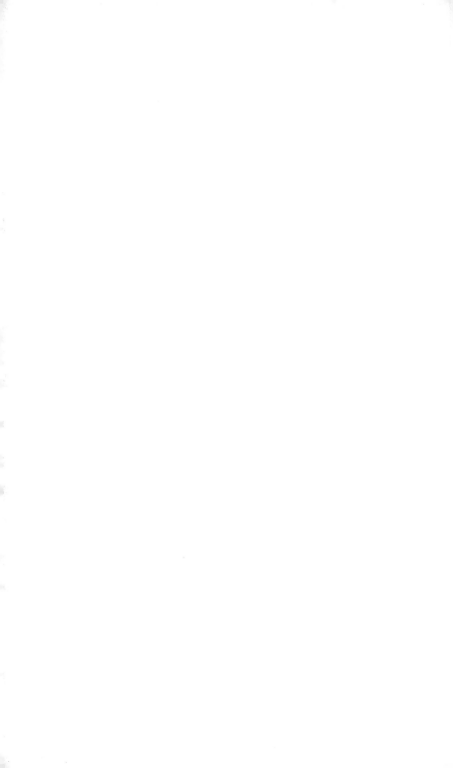

Contents

Contributors

Sean M. Bagshaw, MD
Faculty of Medicine and Dentistry
Division of Critical Care Medicine
University of Alberta
Edmonton, Canada

Ian Baldwin, RN, PhD
Adjunct Professor
Deakin and RMIT Universities
Austin Health
Melbourne, Australia

Ilona Bobek, PhD
Budapest, Hungary

Jorge Cerdá, MD, FACP, FASN
Clinical Professor of Medicine
Department of Medicine
Albany Medical College
Albany, New York

Lakhmir S. Chawla, MD
Associate Professor of Medicine
Department of Medicine
Veterans Affairs Medical Center
Washington, District of Columbia

William R. Clark, MD
Senior Medical Director
Renal Medical Affairs
Baxter Healthcare Corporation
Deerfield, Illinois

Silvia De Rosa

Nigel Fealy, RN, MN, ACCCN
Department of Intensive Care
Austin Hospital
Melbourne, Australia

Kevin W. Finkel, MD, FACP, FASN, FCCM
Professor and Director of Renal
Diseases and Hypertension
University of Texas Health
Science Center
Houston Medical School
Houston, Texas

Francesco Garzotto, PhD
San Bortolo Hospital
Department of Nephrology
Dialysis and Transplantation
International Renal Research
Institute of Vicenza
Vicenza, Italy

Dehua Gong, MD
Research Institute of Nephrology
Jinling Hospital
Nanjing University
Nanjing, China

Zhongping Huang, PhD
Department of Mechanical
Engineering
Widener University
Chester, Pennsylvania

**Sandra L. Kane-Gill, PharmD,
FCCP, FCCM**
Associate Professor of Pharmacy
and Therapeutics
Faculty, School of Pharmacy
Center for Critical Care Nephrology
University of Pittsburgh
University of Pittsburgh
Medical Center
Pittsburgh, Pennsylvania

Joseph E. Kiss, MD
Institute for Transfusion Medicine
University of Pittsburgh School of
Medicine
Pittsburgh, Pennsylvania

Jeffrey J. Letteri, BS
Director
Baxter Healthcare Renal Division
Nantucket, Massachusetts

Michael L. Moritz, MD
Division of Nephrology
Department of Pediatrics
Children's Hospital of Pittsburgh
The University of Pittsburgh School
of Medicine
Pittsburgh, Pennsylvania

**Raghavan Murugan,
MD, FRCP**
Associate Professor of Critical
Care Medicine and Clinical and
Translational Science
Department of Critical Care
Medicine
University of Pittsburgh School
of Medicine
Pittsburgh, Pennsylvania

Mitra K. Nadim, MD
Department of Medicine
University of Southern California
Los Angeles, California

Mauro Neri
International Renal Research
Institute of Vicenza
San Bortolo Hospital
Vicenza, Italy

Paul M. Palevsky, MD
Chief of Renal Section
VA Pittsburgh Healthcare System
Professor of Medicine and Clinical
and Translational Science
University of Pittsburgh School of
Medicine
Pittsburgh, Pennsylvania

Zaccaria Ricci, MD
Pediatric Cardiac Intensive Care Unit
Department of Pediatric Cardiac
Surgery
Bambino Gesù Children's
Hospital, IRCCS
Rome, Italy

Sara Samoni

Ayan Sen, MD, FACEP, FCCP
Consultant and Assistant Professor
of Critical Care and Emergency
Medicine
Mayo Clinic
Phoenix, Arizona

**Kai Singbartl, MB, ChB, PhD,
FRCA, FFA(SA)**
Department of Anesthesiology
Penn State College of Medicine
Hershey, Pennsylvania

Frederick J. Tasota, RN, MSN
UPMC Presbyterian
Pittsburgh, Pennsylvania

Aditya Uppalapati, MD
Department of Medicine
Saint Louis University
Saint Louis, Missouri

Gianluca Villa, MD
International Renal Research
Institute of Vicenza
San Bortolo Hospital
Vicenza, Italy
Department of Health Sciences
Section of Anesthesiology
University of Florence
Florence, Italy

**Kimberly Whiteman,
DNP, RN**
Assistant Professor of Nursing
Co-Director Graduate and
Professional Studies Nursing
Programs
Waynesburg University
Pittsburgh, Pennsylvania

Adrian Wong, PharmD
Resident
University of Pittsburgh School of
Pharmacy
Pittsburgh, Pennsylvania

Alexander Zarbock, MD
Department of Anaesthesiology
Intensive Care and Pain Medicine
University Hospital Münster
Münster, Germany

Part I

Theory

Chapter 1

The Critically Ill Patient with Acute Kidney Injury

Aditya Uppalapati and John A. Kellum

The terms *acute kidney injury* (AKI) and *acute renal failure* (ARF) are not synonymous. Although the term *renal failure* is best reserved for patients who have lost renal function to the point that life can no longer be sustained without intervention, AKI is used to describe the milder as well as severe forms of acute renal dysfunction in patients. Although the analogy is imperfect, the AKI–ARF relationship can be thought of as being similar to the relationship between acute coronary syndrome and ischemic heart failure. AKI is intended to describe the entire spectrum of disease—from being relatively mild to severe. In contrast, renal failure is defined as renal function inadequate to clear the waste products of metabolism despite the absence of or correction of hemodynamic or mechanical causes. Clinical manifestations of renal failure (either acute or chronic) include the following:

- Uremic symptoms (drowsiness, nausea, hiccough, twitching)
- Hyperkalemia
- Hyponatremia
- Metabolic acidosis

Oliguria

Persistent oliguria may be a feature of AKI, but nonoliguric renal failure is not uncommon. Patients may continue to make urine despite an inadequate glomerular filtration. Although prognosis is often better if urine output is maintained, use of diuretics to promote urine output does not seem to improve outcome (and some studies even suggest harm). More important, azotemia (increased serum creatinine [SCrt]) together with oliguria portends a worse prognosis than either sign alone.

Classification

The Kidney Disease Improving Global Outcomes (KDIGO) work group defines AKI as an increase in SCr by 0.3 mg/dL or more (≥26.5 mmol/L)

Table 1.1 KDIGO criteria for staging severity of AKI

Stage	Serum Creatinine Level	Urine Output
1	1.5–1.9 times baseline or (0.3 mg/dL ((26.5 mmol/L) increase	<0.5 mL/kg/h for 6–12 h
2	2.0–2.9 times baseline	<0.5 mL/kg/h for (12 h
3	3.0 times baseline or increase in serum creatinine to (4.0 mg/dL ((353.6 mmol/L) or initiation of renal replacement therapy or, in patients <18 years, decrease in estimated glomerular filtration rate to <35 mL/min per 1.73 m^2	<0.3 mL/kg/h for ≥24 h or anuria for ≥12 h

Source: Kidney Disease: Improving Global Outcomes (KDIGO) Acute Kidney Injury Work Group. KDIGO clinical practice guideline for acute kidney injury. *Kidney Int*. 2012;2(suppl):1–138.

within 48 hours, an increase in SCr to 1.5 times baseline or more, which is known or presumed to have occurred within the prior 7 days, or urine volume less than 0.5 mL/kg/h for 6 hours. AKI is staged for severity as shown in Table 1.1.

Incidence and Etiology of AKI

RIFLE (risk, injury, failure, loss, end-stage kidney disease [ESRD]) criteria developed by the acute dialysis quality initiative and acute kidney injury network (AKIN) criteria developed by an international network of AKI researchers were used to define AKI and its severity. They were based on SCrt level and urine output. Both of these criteria have been well validated in various patient populations. With increasing severity or stage, AKI was associated with increasing mortality. These criteria were adopted by the KDIGO in its AKI clinical practice guideline (Figure 1.1).

Incidence and Progression

AKI occurs in 35% to 65% of intensive care unit (ICU) admissions and 5% to 20% of general hospital admissions. Mortality rates increase significantly with AKI, and most studies show a three- to fivefold increase in the risk of death among patients with AKI compared with patients without AKI. Furthermore, increases in severity of AKI are associated with a stepwise increase in risk of death and need for renal replacement therapy (RRT).

Individuals who survive an AKI hospitalization have a greater likelihood of a recurrent hospital admission compared with those with no evidence of kidney disease (AKI or chronic kidney disease) and are at an increased risk of developing ESRD. Risk factors for developing AKI as defined by KDIGO criteria are presented in Table 1.2.

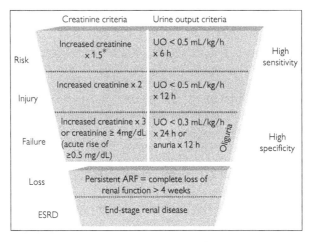

Figure 1.1 The RIFLE cCriteria for diagnosis and staging of acute kidney injury AKI—used to describe three levels of renal impairment (Risk, Injury, Failure) and two clinical outcomes (Loss and End-stage kidney disease). ARF, acute renal failure; UO, urine output. *An alternative proposal is to define "risk" to include any increase in serum creatinine of at least 0.3 mg/dL over 48 hours or less, even if less than a 50% increase.

Source: Bellomo R, Ronco C, Kellum JA, Mehta RL, Palevsky P. Acute renal failure: definition, outcome measures, animal models, fluid therapy and information technology needs: the Second International Consensus Conference of the Acute Dialysis Quality Initiative (ADQI) Group. *Crit Care*. 2004;8:R204–R212. Used with permission.

Table 1.2 Risk factors for developing AKI as defined by KDIGO criteria

Increasing age, especially older than 65 years	Surgical admissions more likely than medical admissions*
Female gender	Cardiac surgery
Black race*	Sepsis
Dehydration or volume depletion	Radio contrast media
Hypoalbuminemia	Shock
Preexisting chronic kidney disease	Cancer
Diabetes mellitus	Genetic factors/polymorphisms*
Cardiac dysfunction (CAD, LVEF <35%)	Drugs: NSAIDs, ACE-I,* diuretics, cyclosporine, tacrolimus, penicillin, aminoglycosides
Chronic obstructive pulmonary disease*	
Mechanical ventilation	
Chronic liver disease	
Critical illness, trauma	

ACE-I, angiotensin-converting enzyme inhibitor; CAD, coronary artery disease; LVEF, left ventricular ejection fraction; NSAIDs, nonsteroidal anti-inflammatory drugs.

*Evidence is inconclusive.

Etiology of AKI

Clinical features may suggest the cause of AKI and dictate further investigation. AKI is common in the critically ill, especially in patients with sepsis and other forms of systemic inflammation (e.g., major surgery, trauma, burns), but other causes must be considered.

Volume-Responsive AKI

It is estimated that as many as 50% of cases of AKI are "fluid responsive," and the first step in managing any case of AKI is to ensure appropriate fluid resuscitation. However, volume overload is a key factor contributing to the mortality attributable to AKI, so ongoing fluid administration to nonfluid-responsive patients is discouraged.

Sepsis-Induced AKI

Sepsis is a primary cause or contributing factor in more than 50% of cases of AKI, which includes cases severe enough to require RRT. Patients with sepsis, including those outside the ICU, develop AKI at rates as high as 40%. Incidence increases with the severity of sepsis. Sepsis-induced AKI can develop in patients with normal, decreased, as well as increased renal blood flow. In sepsis, the kidney often has a normal histological appearance.

Hypotension

Hypotension is an important risk factor for AKI, and many patients with AKI have sustained at least one episode of hypotension. Treating fluid-responsive AKI with fluid resuscitation is clearly an important step, but many patients also require vasoactive therapy (e.g., norepinephrine) to maintain arterial blood pressure. Despite a common belief among many practitioners, norepinephrine does not increase the risk of AKI compared with dopamine, and renal blood flow actually increases with norepinephrine in animal models of sepsis.

Postoperative AKI

Risk factors of postoperative AKI include hypovolemia, hypotension, major abdominal surgery, and sepsis. Surgical procedures (particularly gynecological) may be complicated by damage to the lower urinary tract with an obstructive nephropathy. Abdominal aortic aneurysm surgery may be associated with renal arterial disruption. Cardiac surgery may be associated with atheroembolism, hemolysis, and sustained periods of reduced arterial pressure as well as systemic inflammation.

Other Causes

- *Nephrotoxins*: May cause renal failure via direct tubular injury, interstitial nephritis, or renal tubular obstruction. In patients with AKI, all potential nephrotoxins should be withdrawn.

- *Rhabdomyolysis*: Suggested by myoglobinuria and increased creatine kinase levels in patients who have experienced a crush injury, coma, or seizures. Often, elevated liver transaminases—aspartate aminotransferase > alanine aminotransferase—are also noted as a result of muscular injury.
- *Glomerular disease*: Red cell casts, hematuria, proteinuria, and systemic features (e.g., hypertension, purpura, arthralgia, vasculitis) are all suggestive of glomerular disease. Renal biopsy or specific blood tests (e.g., Goodpasture's syndrome, vasculitis) are required to confirm diagnosis and guide appropriate treatment.
- *Hemolytic uremic syndrome*: Suggested by hemolysis, uremia, thrombocytopenia, and neurological abnormalities
- *Crystal nephropathy*: Suggested by the presence of crystals in the urinary sediment. Microscopic examination of the crystals confirms the diagnosis (e.g., urate, oxalate). Release of purines and urate are responsible for ARF in tumor lysis syndrome.
- *Renovascular disorders*: Loss of vascular supply may be diagnosed by renography. Complete loss of arterial supply may occur in abdominal trauma or aortic disease (particularly dissection). More commonly, the arterial supply is compromised in part (e.g., renal artery stenosis) and blood flow is further reduced by hemodynamic instability or locally via drug therapy (e.g., nonsteroidal anti-inflammatory drugs [NSAIDs], angiotensin-converting enzyme inhibitors). Renal vein obstruction may be a result of thrombosis or external compression (e.g., raised intra-abdominal pressure).
- *Abdominal compartment syndrome*: Suggested by oliguria, a firm abdomen on physical examination, and increased airway pressures (secondary to upward pressure on the diaphragms). Diagnosis is likely when sustained, increased intra-abdominal pressures (bladder pressure measured at end expiration in the supine position) exceed 25 mmHg. However, abdominal compartment syndrome may occur with intra-abdominal pressures as low as 10 mmHg.

Nephrotoxins

Box 1.1 lists some medications that can be nephrotoxic. In addition, aminoglycosides, NSAIDs, allopurinol, furosemide, sulfonamides, thiazides, pentamidine, amphotericin, organic solvents, Paraquat, herbal medicines, and heavy metals are also nephrotoxic.

Evaluation of AKI

Evaluation of AKI is based on clinical history, physical examination, laboratory results, and assessment of hemodynamics and volume status. Newer

Box 1.1 Common Nephrotoxic Drugs

- Antibiotics (penicillins, cephalosporins, sulfa, rifampin, quinolones)
- Diuretics (furosemide, bumetanide, thiazides)
- NSAIDS (including selective COX-2 inhibitors)
- Allopurinol
- Cimetidine (rarely other H2 blockers)
- Proton pump inhibitors (omeprazole, lansoprazole)
- Indinavir
- 5-Aminosalicylates

Table 1.3 Evaluation of AKI

Clinical history and examination

Conduct an ultrasound of the bladder and kidneys if suspected retention, obstruction, hydronephrosis.

Insert Foley catheter if needed and check for patency; flush catheter.

If abdomen is distended and tense, check bladder pressure.

Clinical Assessment	Urine Analysis		
Hemodynamics		Prerenal	Intrinsic Renal
• Mean arterial pressure, heart rate	Osmolality (mOsm/L)	>500	<350
• Volume status and central venous pressure, examination, chest radiograph	Sodium (mmol/L)	<20	>40
	Fractional excretion sodium (%)	<1	>2
• Echocardiogram, right ventricular and left ventricular function	Urea (%)	<35	>35
Fluid responsiveness	Microscopy	Hyaline casts	Muddy brown: ARF trial network (ATN)
• Passive leg raise test, stroke volume variation, pulse pressure variation, velocity time integral variability, inferior vena cava distensibility index			Bacteria, white blood cells: pyelonephritis
			Eosinophils: interstitial nephritis
			Red blood cell casts: evaluate for vasculitis, glomerulonephritis
			Red blood cells: consider renal artery or vein occlusion
Biomarkers	Urinary [TIMP-2]•[IGFBP7]: >0.3, high risk; >2.0, very high (40%–50%) chance of developing stage 2/3 acute kidney infection in the next 12–24 h; plasma/urine NGAL, interleukin 18, KIM-1, L-FABP		

biomarkers are also gaining strength in the early detection and evaluation of AKI. Urine analysis can be suggestive but not diagnostic of AKI etiology (Table 1.3).

Management of AKI

Identification and correction of reversible causes of AKI is critical. All cases require careful attention to fluid management and nutritional support.

Urinary Tract Obstruction

Lower tract obstruction requires the insertion of a catheter (suprapubic if there is a urethral disruption) to allow decompression. Ureteric obstruction requires urinary tract decompression by nephrostomy or stent. A massive diuresis is common after decompression, so it is important to ensure adequate circulating volume to prevent secondary AKI.

Hemodynamic Management

Fluid-responsive AKI may be reversible in its early stage. However, volume overload is a key factor contributing to the mortality attributable to AKI, so ongoing fluid administration to nonfluid-responsive patients is discouraged. In severe cases, fluid resuscitation may be guided by functional hemodynamic monitoring, and parameters such as stroke volume variation, pulse pressure variation, velocity time integral variability, inferior vena cava distensibility index, and the passive leg raise test can help guide fluid responsiveness. After assessing fluid status and volume responsiveness, necessary inotrope or vasopressor support should be started to ensure tissue perfusion.

Glomerular Disease

Specific therapy in the form of immunosuppressive drugs may be useful after diagnosis has been confirmed.

Interstitial Nephritis

Acute interstitial nephritis most often results from drug therapy. However, other causes include autoimmune disease and infection (e.g., Legionella, leptospirosis, *Streptococcus*, cytomegalovirus). Numerous drugs have been implicated, but the most common ones are as listed in Box 1.1.

Table 1.4 Clinical consequences of AKI

System	Mechanisms	Complications
Electrolyte disturbances	• Hyponatremia • Hyperkalemia	• Central nervous system (see Nervous System) • Malignant arrhythmias
Acid–base (decreased chloride excretion, accumulation of organic anions such as PO4, decreased albumin, buffering)	• Downregulation of beta receptors, increased inducible nitric oxide synthase • Hyperchloremia • Impairment of insulin resistance • Innate immunity	• Decreased cardiac output, blood pressure • Lung, intestinal injury, decreased gut barrier function • Hyperglycemia, increased protein breakdown • See below
Cardiovascular	• Volume overload	• Congestive heart failure • Secondary hypertension
Pulmonary	• Volume overload, decreased oncotic pressure • Infiltration and activation of lung neutrophils by cytokines • Uremia	• Pulmonary edema, pleural effusions • Acute lung injury • Pulmonary hemorrhage
Gastrointestinal	• Volume overload • Gut ischemia and reperfusion • injury	• Abdominal compartment syndrome • Acute gastric and duodenal ulcer bleeding, impaired nutrient absorption
Immune	• Decreased clearance of oxidant stress • Tissue edema • White cell dysfunction	• Increased risk of infection • Delayed wound healing
Hematological	• Decreased synthesis of RBCs, increased destruction of RBCs, blood loss • Decreased production of erythropoietin, von Willebrand factor	• Anemia • Bleeding
Nervous system	• Secondary hepatic failure, malnutrition, altered drug metabolism • Hyponatremia, acidosis • Uremia	• Altered mental status • Seizures, impaired consciousness, coma • Myopathy, neuropathy: prolonged length on mechanical ventilation
Pharmacokinetics and dynamics	• Increased volume of distribution • Decreased availability, albumin binding, elimination	• Drug toxicity or underdosing

RBC, red blood cell.

Urine sediment may reveal white cells, red cells, and white cell casts. Eosinophiluria is present in about two-thirds of cases, and specificity for interstitial nephritis is only about 80%. Other causes of AKI in which eosinophiluria is relatively common are rapidly progressive glomerulonephritis and renal atheroemboli. Discontinuation of the potential causative agent is a mainstay of therapy.

Abdominal Compartment Syndrome

Baseline blood pressure and abdominal wall compliance influence the amount of intra-abdominal pressure that can be tolerated. Enteral decompression with nasogastric or rectal tubes, percutaneous drainage to remove intra-abdominal fluid, and a brief trial of neuromuscular blockade might help as a temporizing method. However, surgical decompression is the only definitive therapy and should be undertaken before irreversible end-organ damage occurs.

Renal Replacement Therapy

CRRT forms the mainstay of replacement therapy in critically ill patients who often cannot tolerate standard hemodialysis because of hemodynamic instability. Hybrid techniques (discussed in Chapter 25) may be reasonable alternatives in settings in which CRRT cannot be accomplished, but outcome data are limited. Peritoneal dialysis is not usually sufficient. Mortality in the setting of ARF in the critically ill is high (40%–60%). Recent studies suggest that sustained renal failure or incomplete renal recovery is more common than previously thought (as many as 50% of survivors do not return to baseline renal function after an episode of ARF).

Clinical Consequences of AKI

Until recently, it was assumed that patients with AKI died, not because of AKI itself, but because of their underlying disease. Several studies, however, have documented a substantial mortality attributable to AKI after controlling for other variables, including chronic illness and severity of underlying acute illness. Table 1.4 lists some of the more important clinical consequences of AKI.

Key References

Kellum JA. Acute kidney injury. Crit Care Med. 2008;36:S141–S145.

1. Kidney Disease: Improving Global Outcomes (KDIGO) Acute Kidney Injury Work Group. KDIGO Clinical Practice Guideline for Acute Kidney Injury. *Kidney Int.er.*, Suppl. 2012;2(suppl):1–138.

2. Kellum JA. Acute Kidney Injury. Crit Care Med. 2008;36:S141–S145.

3. Uchino S, Kellum JA, Bellomo R, et al. Acute renal failure in critically ill patients: a multinational, multicenter study. JAMA. 2005;294:813–818.

Chapter 2

History and Rationale for Continuous Renal Replacement Therapy

Ilona Bobek and Claudio Ronco

Medical Demand/Necessity for Continuous Renal Replacement Therapy

Clinical Picture of Acute Renal Failure Changed during the 1980s

Underlying diseases leading to acute renal failure (ARF) were severe sepsis and occurred frequently after abortions before, whereas its epidemiological pattern and the involvement of other organs became more and more common after the 1990s.

- The cases of isolated (purely nephrological) ARF decreased as a result of early diagnosis and better prophylaxis.
- More patients received increasingly extensive operations and survived serious accidents.
- The number of patients in the intensive care unit (ICU) increased significantly.
- In the ICU, patients had a longer stay with the possibility of better outcomes.

Pathogenesis of ARF Changed

The main factors recently responsible for ARF include the following:

- Shock
- Perfusion disturbances
- Hypoxia

Chronology/Cornerstones of Continuous Renal Replacement Therapy

1960 The idea for continuous renal replacement therapy (CRRT) was born, but supplies and technology were not available. Most of ARF was treated with Peritoneal dialysis (PD), because hemodialysis (HD) was difficult to perform and it was not tolerated by ICU patients.

1970s Henderson played an important role in the technical groundwork for hemofiltration. Isolated ultrafiltration (UF) and use of convection for solute removal was established experimentally.

1977 First description of an arteriovenous hemofiltration technique by Kramer and colleagues in Göttingen, Germany.

After a vascular catheter was placed accidentally into the femoral artery raised the idea to use the systemic arteriovenous pressure difference in an extracorporeal circuit to generate the ultrafiltrate providing an effective method for elimination of both fluid and solutes. Heparin could be added before and fluid could be reinfused after the filter. Continuous arteriovenous hemofiltration (CAVH) was soon accepted worldwide in ICUs (Figure 2.1).

Advantages of CAVH
- Hemodynamic stability over conventional HD at that time
- Simple
- No necessity for blood pump
- Continuous physiological fluid removal

Limitations of CAVH
- Low efficiency compared with HD
- Reduced clearance capacity in the presence of high catabolic states

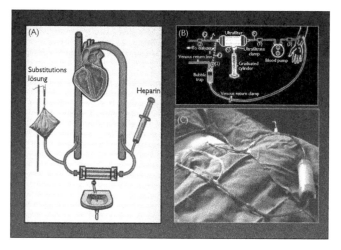

Figure 2.1 (A, B) The concept, by Peter Kramer and Lee Henderson, of continuous filtration. (C) The first patient treated with continuous arteriovenous hemofiltration in Vicenza, Italy, in 1978.

- Additional intermittent HD or hemofiltration (HF) often necessary
- Complications associated with arterial access (indwelling catheters, thrombosis)
- Reliance on arterial pressure to pump blood through the circuit
- Danger of balancing errors
- Necessity for continuous supervision by the staff

1979 Continuous venous–venous hemofiltration (CVVH) was first used in ARF after cardiac surgery in Cologne, Germany. Any desired filtrate volume could be arranged, and uremia was controlled. A pump, control, and balancing system became necessary (Figure 2.2).

1980s Numerous technical and methodical improvements in CRRT have contributed.

Changes in Arteriovenous Technique
- Different types of catheters to obtain adequate blood flow
- Shorter blood line with no gadgets to reduce resistance
- Positioning the collecting bag to apply a negative pressure
- Optimization of treatment parameters, concept of filtration fraction
- Changes in filter geometry and in the structure of fiber (An entire family of hemofilters was created to fulfill hemodynamic requirements.)
- An increase in efficiency as a result of dialysis fluid being filtered through the external port of the filter; Continuous arterio-venous hemodialysis (CAVHD) implemented
- Combination of hemofiltration and hemodialysis; Continuous arterio-venous hemodiafiltration (CAVHDF) was performed

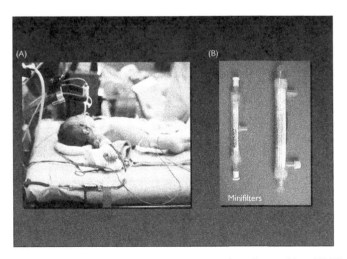

Figure 2.2 A typical system for continuous venous–venous hemofiltration (Hospal BM32).

Pump-Driven Venous–Venous Techniques
Replaced Arteriovenous Techniques

- Blood pump to increase efficiency further; CVVH introduced
- Double-lumen catheters used in jugular vein
- Highly permeable polysulfone, polyacrylonitrile, and polyamide membranes developed with a cutoff between 15,000 Da and 50,000 Da.
- Bicarbonate–buffer solutions became available
- New anticoagulation methods established, even for patients at high risk of bleeding

1982 Use of CAVH in ICU patients approved by the Food and Drug Administration in the United States.

1984 The first neonate was treated with CAVH in the world occurred in Vicenza, Italy (Figure 2.3).

1990–2000 Establishment of new technologies, modalities, and adequate dose of CRRT:

- Adoptive technology
- Machines created specifically for CRRT (Figure 2.4)
- Different therapies chosen based on the needs of the patient
- Progression of dose delivery and prescription

CRRT is achievable in most ICUs worldwide.

2000 Multiorgan support therapy (MOST)

Patients do not die of ARF but of multiorgan failure. The probability of death correlates directly with the number of failing organs, other than the

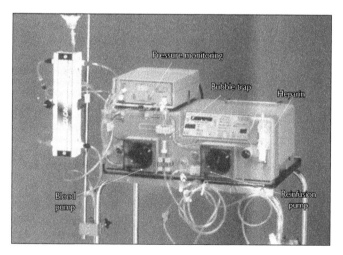

Figure 2.3 The first neonate treated in the world with continuous arteriovenous hemofiltration and a special minifilter in Vicenza, Italy, in 1984.

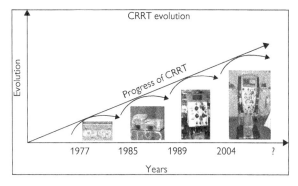

Figure 2.4 The evolution of continuous renal replacement therapy (CRRT) technology throughout the years. The case of a single company.

kidney and the severity of physiological disorders. The proper goal of extracorporeal blood purification in the ICU should be MOST. Treatment should not directed at various organs as separate entities (Figure 2.5); it should be integrated and patient directed. Therefore, a wide range of supportive therapies in sepsis and liver failure were established, such as high-volume hemofiltration (HVHF), coupled plasma filtration and adsorption (CPFA), bio-artificial livers, and endotoxin removal strategies.

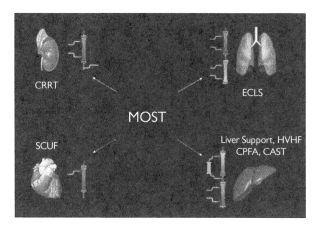

Figure 2.5 The concept of multiorgan support therapy (MOST). Blood can be circulated by a platform through different filtration/adsorption systems, leading to removal of specific compounds and support to different failing organs. CAST, XXXXX; CPFA, coupled plasma filtration adsorption; CRRT, continuous renal replacement therapy; ECLS, extracorporeal lung support system; HVHF, high-volume hemofiltration; SCUF, slow continuous ultrafiltration.

2000 Founding of the Acute Dialysis Quality Initiative (ADQI)

The ADQI is an ongoing process that seeks to produce evidence-based recommendations for the prevention and management of acute kidney injury (AKI) and on different issues concerning acute renal replacement therapy (RRT). The following goals have been achieved:

• Definition and classification of ARF (RIFLE criteria, acute kidney injury network (AKIN))
• Practice guidelines adopted in clinical practice (cardiac surgery-associated AKI)

Recent interest focuses on the timing of treatment initiation on patient survival, dose of RRT, fluid management, and the effect of RRT modality on recovery of renal function in ARF.

Future processes involve the online preparation of reinfusion fluids during high-volume hemofiltration, studies on microfluidics and technology for plasma separation, miniaturized technologies, bio-artificial devices, new sorbent techniques, nanotechnology, and wearable/transportable devices.

RRT has evolved from the concept of needing to treat the dysfunction of a single organ (the kidney). However, CRRT has also opened the door to the concept of MOST. Future treatment requires one multifunctional machine with a user-friendly interface, flexibility in parameters, and prescription such that it can be used to respond to different medical needs using different disposable layouts. The new generation of machines should be usable by different operators in different hospitals and settings.

The numerous ADQI meetings organized throughout the years have dealt with specific topics that represent the core interest of the scientific community dealing with AKI. In particular, the following conferences were organized that led to milestone publications (prefaced by an asterisk in the list of key references): CRRT, New York, 2000; AKI Research, Vicenza, Italy, 2002; Non-renal Blood Purification, Miami, Florida, 2003; Prevention of AKI, Vicenza, Italy, 2004; Fluid Management in AKI, Tambor, Costa Rica, 2007; AKI in Cardiac Surgery, Vicenza, Italy, 2007; Cardio Renal Syndrome, Venice, Italy, 2008; Hepatorenal Syndrome, Kauai, Hawaii, 2010; Toxicology, Denver, Colorado, 2010; Biomarkers, Dublin, Ireland, 2011; Cardio Renal Pathophysiology, Venice, Italy, 2012; Fluids Reloaded, London, United Kingdom, 2013; and AKI Research Review, Charlottesville, 2014.

2000–2015 Large Studies on Dose and survival

After the publication of the first study on the effects of treatment dose on survival, other large studies were conducted and large databases were collected to analyze the effects of treatment modality and dose of therapy. The

AKIN also facilitated studies in the area of ARRT and AKI. These studies led to the definition of a certain standard of care in the field of RRT for the critically ill patient.

2013 The Kidney Disease Improving Global Outcomes Guidelines

Another milestone is represented by the publication of AKI guidelines. Numerous studies published throughout the years have led to a specific focus on standard of care and quality of treatment delivery. In particular, the Kidney Disease Improving Global Outcomes work group published the AKI guidelines, offering a distillation of the available evidence and consequent possible recommendations.

Key References

Bellomo R, Palevsky PM, Bagshaw SM, et al. Recent trials in critical care nephrology. *Contrib Nephrol.* 2010;165:299–309.

Henderson LW. Peritoneal ultrafiltration dialysis: enhanced urea transfer using hypertonic peritoneal fluid. *JCI.* 1966;45:950–961.

Henderson LW, Besarab A, Michaels A, Bluemle LW. Blood purification by ultrafiltration and fluid replacement (diafiltration). *Trans ASAIO.* 1967;13:216.

Kellum JA, Lameire N, KDIGO AKI guideline work group. Diagnosis, evaluation, and management of acute kidney injury: a KDIGO summary (part 1). *Crit Care.* 2013;17(1):204.

Kellum JA, Mehta R, Angus DC, et al. The first international consensus conference on continuous renal replacement therapy. *Kidney Int.* 2002;62:1855–1863.

Kramer P, Wigger W, Rieger J, Matthaei D, Scheler F. Arterio-venous hemofiltration: *a new simple method for treatment of overhydrated patients resistant to diuretic. Klin Woeschr.* 1977;55:1121–1122.

McCullough PA, Kellum JA, Mehta RL, Murray PT, Ronco C, eds. ADQI Consensus on AKI biomarkers and cardiorenal syndromes. *Contrib Nephrol.* 2013;182:1–4.

Ronco C, Bellomo R. Acute renal failure and multiple organ dysfunction in the ICU: from renal replacement therapy (RRT) to multiple organ support therapy (MOST). *Int J Artif Organs.* 2002;25:733–747.

Ronco C, Bellomo R, Brendolan A, et al. Effect of different doses in continuous veno–venous haemofiltration on outcomes of acute renal failure: a prospective randomized trial. *Lancet.* 2000;355:26–30.

Sieberth HG, History and development of continuous renal replacement (CRRT). *Critical Care Nephology.* 1161-1167, Dordrecht: Kluwer Academic Publishers, 1998.

Vesconi S, Cruz DN, Fumagalli R, et al. Delivered dose of renal replacement therapy and mortality in critically ill patients with acute kidney injury. *Crit Care.* 2009;13(2):R57.

Chapter 3

Nomenclature for Renal Replacement Therapy in Acute Kidney Injury

Mauro Neri, Jorge Cerdá, Francesco Garzotto, Gianluca Villa, and Claudio Ronco

The management of critically ill patients with acute kidney injury (AKI) requiring renal replacement therapy (RRT) demands a multidisciplinary approach. When nephrologists, intensivists, and nurses gather at the bedside to decide on management strategies and to implement treatment, they make a series of decisions. The apparent simplicity of this process belies an enormous degree of complexity, which requires profound expertise, a thorough understanding of different treatment options, and optimal timing (Box 3.1).

The terminology used to describe the different modalities of RRT is often confusing and continuously evolving. In this chapter, we provide an updated consensus nomenclature that helps navigate this complex field, primarily aiming to attain a shared language among all parties involved. To facilitate comprehension and progress, we expect that industry will also adopt this standard terminology.

We describe the basic principles underlying RRT technologies and the application of those principles to direct patient care. The aim of this chapter is to focus on the basic aspects and applications of continuous renal replacement therapies (CRRT) that are most often used in the treatment of the critically ill patient with severe AKI. We provide a thorough description of the CRRT hardware and disposables, the solutes and fluid transport mechanisms across membranes, and the different prescribing modalities.

To ensure a complete review of the RRT nomenclature used in the intensive care unit (ICU), we screened the literature of the past 25 years and implemented previous taxonomy efforts. We completed an extensive literature search for documents published in English from January 1990 to date. Keywords included *continuous renal replacement therapy* and *dialysis, hemofiltration, convection, diffusion, ultrafiltration, dose, blood purification, renal support, multiorgan dysfunction*, and their relative MeSH (Medical Subject Headings) terms. We decided not to include the topics *arteriovenous treatments* and *vascular access*. Abstracts of 707 articles were screened, and more than 300 papers were read and analyzed extensively. Each definition has received the consensus of at least two of the three reviewers (MN, FG, and GV).

Box 3.1 Considerations When Prescribing Renal Replacement Therapy for AKI

Consideration	Components	Application
Modality	Intermittent hemodialysis	Daily, every other day; hybrid therapies
	Continuous renal replacement therapies	Multiple varieties
	Peritoneal dialysis	Multiple varieties
Membrane characteristics	Geometric and performance characteristics; convection, diffusion	Dialysis, hemoperfusion, hemadsorption
Biocompatibility		
Dialyzer performance	Efficiency, intensity, and efficacy	
	Flux	
Dialysis delivery	Timing of initiation	Early, late
	Adequacy of dialysis	Dialysis dose
		Prescription vs. delivery

Source: Modified from Cerda J, Ronco C. Modalities of continuous renal replacement therapy: technical and clinical considerations. *Semin Dial*. 2009;22(2):114–122.

Hardware, Devices and Disposables

CRRT "hardware" includes the machine and dedicated disposables. Knowledge of the nomenclature and the functions of the whole machine and its main components is extremely important, not only for the nurses or technicians who are the main users of the device, but also for clinicians who make the prescription and manage patient care. In this section, we include relevant nursing procedures and their specific terminology.

The disposables (single-use components of the extracorporeal circuit) are specific for every machine and are usually designed for a specific treatment modality. The main disposables and color codes that should mark each tubing line are listed in Box 3.2.

During a CRRT treatment, the filter is the key disposable where blood is effectively depurated. Historically, the designation filter describes the entire depurative extracorporeal device system (e.g., membranes, housing). However, a more accurate use of specific terms should restrict the designation to the devices that purify blood by different transport mechanisms and modalities. In particular, the terms *hemofilter, dialyzer* (or *hemodialyzer*), and *diafilter* (or *hemodiafilter*) should be used if exclusively convective, diffusive, or diffusive plus convective modalities are applied, respectively. *Plasma filter* is defined as a specific filter that permits the separation of plasma components

Box 3.2 Main Disposables and Their Components with Associated Color Code in a CRRT Extracorporeal Circuit

Tubes	Arterial line (red)		Segment connecting the patient's arterial vascular access to the dialyzer
		Segment for pressure measure (upstream arterial pump)	Segment of the arterial line connected to the arterial pressure sensor
		Pump segment line	Segment inserted between the rotor and the stator of the blood pump
		Arterial air removal chamber	Allowance of light air bubble removal before the blood entrance into the dialyzer
		Segment for pressure measure (downstream arterial pump)	Segment of the arterial line connected to the prefilter pressure sensor
	Venous line (dark blue)		Segment connecting the dialyzer to the patient's venous vascular access
		Segment for pressure measure	Segment of the venous line connected to the venous pressure sensor
		Venous air removal chamber	Allowance of light air bubble removal before the blood returns to the patient
	Effluent/ ultrafiltrate line (yellow)		Segment that allows the flow of wasting fluids coming from the dialyzer
		Pump segment line	Segment inserted between the rotor and the stator of the effluent/ ultrafiltrate pump
		Segment for pressure measure	Segment of the effluent line connected to the effluent/ultrafiltrate pressure sensor
	Dialysate line (green)		Segment that allows the flow of incoming dialysate into the dialyzer
		Pump segment line	Segment inserted between the rotor and the stator of the dialysate pump
		Segment for pressure measure (if present)	Segment of the dialysate line connected to the dialysate pressure sensor
		Heater line	Segment of the dialysate line placed in contact with the heater
	Replacement line (purple or light blue)		Segment that allows the flow of replacement fluid into the arterial and/ or venous lines
		Pump segment line	Segment inserted between the rotor and the stator of the replacement pump
		Segment for pressure measure (if present)	Segment of the replacement line connected to the replacement pressure sensor

(continued)

Box 3.2 Continued

		Heater line	Segment of the replacement line placed in contact with the heater
	Preblood line (orange)		Segment that allows the flow of specific fluids into the arterial line before the blood pump
		Pump segment line	Segment inserted between the rotor and the stator of the pre-blood pump
		Segment for pressure measure (if present)	Segment of the pre-blood line connected to the pre-blood pressure sensor
	Anticoagulant and specific antagonists line		Segments connecting the anticoagulant/ specific antagonist bag or pump to the main blood circuit
		Citrate line	Segment for citrate infusion (i.e., pre-blood line)
		Heparin line	Segment connecting the heparin syringe pump to the arterial line
		Specific antagonist line	Segment connecting the specific antagonist syringe pump to the venous line
Filter	Fiber (membranes)		Every fiber and hollow of cylindrical shape; allowance of fluid and solute transport phenomena through their porous semipermeable surface
	Bundle		Entire number of fibers inside the housing
	Housing		Plastic casing containing a single membrane fiber bundle
		Blood inflow port	Entrance port of arterial blood
		Blood outflow port	Exit port of venous blood
		Dialysate inflow port	Entrance port of fresh dialysate
		Effluent/ultrafiltrate outflow port	Exit port of waste solution
	Potting		Polyurethane component fixing the bundle within the housing and embedding the bundle at both ends of the dialyzer

from cellular elements. Sorbents are particular filters where adsorption is the only depurative modality. Nowadays, the only available type of CRRT filter able to perform diffusive and/or convective transport is shaped as a collection of parallel "hollow fibers."

These devices can be identified mainly by membrane geometrics and performance characteristics. A thorough description of the characteristics of the dialysis membrane is included in the Appendix.

Mechanisms of Solute and Fluid Transport

Solute transport occurs mainly by two phenomena: convection and diffusion. The only mechanism that determines fluid transport across semipermeable membranes is ultrafiltration. In addition, adsorption influences solute removal and the two former processes.

Ultrafiltration and Convection

Ultrafiltration is the phenomenon of transport of plasma water (solvent) through a semipermeable membrane driven by a pressure gradient between blood and dialysate/ultrafiltrate compartments. Ultrafiltration is influenced by intrinsic properties of the membrane, such as K_{UF}, and operating parameters (e.g., transmembrane pressure). Quantitatively, the ultrafiltration is defined by the ultrafiltration rate:

$$Q_{UF} = K_{UF} \cdot TMP,$$

where Q_{UF} is Ultrafiltration flow rate, K_{UF} is Filtration Coefficient, and TMP is Transmembrane Pressure.

Convection is the process by which solutes pass through the membrane pores dragged by fluid movement (ultrafiltration) caused by a hydrostatic or osmotic transmembrane pressure gradient.

The convective flux (J_c) of a solute depends on the Q_{UF}, the solute concentration in blood water (C_b), and the solute (SC):

$$J_c = Q_{UF} \cdot C_b \cdot SC.$$

Compared with diffusive transport, convective transport permits the removal of higher molecular weight solutes than diffusive transport.

Diffusion

Diffusion is a process during which molecules move across a membrane in all directions. Statistically, this movement results in the passage of solutes from a more concentrated to a less concentrated area until equilibrium concentration between the two sites is reached. The concentration gradient ($C_1 - C_2 = dc$) is the driving force; the theoretical unidirectional solute diffusive flux (J_d) through a semipermeable membrane follows Fick's law of diffusivity and depends on the surface area (A) and the diffusivity coefficient (D) of the solute, and is inversely proportional to the compartments distance (dx):

$$J_d = -DA\left(\frac{dc}{dx}\right).$$

The diffusivity coefficient D can be approximated by the Stokes-Einstein equation:

$$D = \frac{k_B T}{6\pi\mu R},$$

where k_B is the Boltzmann constant, T is the absolute temperature, μ is the viscosity of the medium, and R is the effective radius of the molecules. Based on the assumption that most molecules are globular and their effective radius is proportional to the cube root of their molecular weight, D is greater for smaller molecular weight solutes.

Adsorption

Adsorption is an extracorporeal process during which hydrophobic compounds in plasma or blood (in particular, peptides and proteins) bind to the membrane structure or to other adsorbed substances such as charcoal, resins, gels, proteins, or monoclonal antibodies. Because this mechanism occurs at the pores more than at the membrane surface, a more open pore structure (typical of high-flux membranes) has a greater adsorption potential. The characteristics that influence protein–membrane interaction are typical for each protein (e.g., dimension, charge, structure) and for each particular membrane (e.g., porosity, composition, hydrophobicity, surface potential). The adsorption affinity of certain high-flux synthetic membranes for proteins and peptides can be very high, making this process the main mechanism of toxin removal

Modalities of Extracorporeal RRT

Hemodialysis

The main mechanism of solute removal in hemodialysis (HD) is diffusion, which is especially effective in the removal of small solutes. HD involves the use of a hemodialyzer, in which blood and an appropriate dialysate solution circulate countercurrent or co-current. A countercurrent configuration is preferred because the average concentration gradient is kept higher along the whole length of the dialyzer. Conversely, a co-current configuration guarantees better stability and control of hydrodynamic conditions, and better air removal during the priming phase. High-flux dialyzers can achieve significant convective transport. This modality is called *high-flux hemodialysis*.

Hemofiltration

Hemofiltration is an exclusively ultrafiltration/convection treatment during which no dialysis fluid is used. Infusion of a sterile solution into the blood circuit replaces the reduced plasma volume and reduces the solute concentration. Infusion of a sterile solution (replacement fluid) can replace the filtered volume totally or partially. Replacement fluid can be infused prefilter (predilution) or postfilter (postdilution). Highly permeable membranes are used. The achievable ultrafiltration (and convective) volume removal over time depends on the membrane K_{UF}. In terms of solute clearance, postdilution is more efficient than the predilution modality, but it can lead more easily to membrane fouling as a result of hemoconcentration.

Hemodiafiltration

Hemodiafiltration combines both HD and hemofiltration whereby the mechanisms involved in solute removal are both diffusive and convective. Dialysate flow configuration can be countercurrent or cocurrent. Because this modality uses very highly permeable membranes, adequate infusion of sterile solution must replace the removed volume, which can be infused prefilter or postfilter. The magnitude of fluid removal depends on whether volume replacement is partial or complete.

Isolated Ultrafiltration

The main goal of ultrafiltration is to remove fluid by convection using highly permeable membranes without volume replacement. Ultrafiltration removes solutes in terms of mass, rather than concentration. As a result of "solvent drag," small solutes are removed minimally, and the concentration of these small solutes in the ultrafiltrate is equal to that of plasma.

Hemoperfusion

In hemoperfusion, blood circulates through a column containing specific sorbents; adsorption is the only removal mechanism. Usually combined with other modalities, hemoperfusion is used to remove specific lipid-soluble substances, toxins, or poisons for which the device is produced to remove, including, for example, certain bacterial toxins or cytokines in sepsis, uremic toxins, mediators of hepatic encephalopathy, or abnormal proteins in dialysis-related amyloidosis. Depending on the characteristics of the membrane, drugs or drug metabolites may also be removed.

Fluids, Volumes, and Flows

Solute transport during extracorporeal treatments depends strictly on operating conditions involving blood flow, dialysate, net ultrafiltration, and replacement flow rates designed to achieve a desired clearance performance. Definitions of the variables involved in fluid volumes and flows are defined in the glossary.

Volume Management and Fluid Balance

In critically ill patients treated with CRRT, management of fluid balance is one of the main goals of treatment. Fluid management prescription during CRRT must take into account primarily the volume status of the patient and the patient's hemodynamic stability, as well as the underlying disease.

Potential mistakes in fluid management include errors in the prescription, operator errors when inputting treatment parameters, or delivery errors resulting from machine malfunction. Clinical complications resulting from an incorrect fluid exchange are important but are frequently underestimated. Discrepancies between prescribed and delivered volumes must also be highlighted.

A "machine fluid balance error" can influence significantly the total volume exchanged. Other factors must also be taken into account, including nutritional support, oral fluid/food intake, blood transfusions, drugs/anticoagulant infusion, diuresis, surgical drains, and other specific clinical conditions. Patient weight and, consequently, the fluid balance must be monitored continuously using a bed scale.

In clinical practice, the CRRT prescription refers only to fluid removal; fluid balance error can be defined as either positive or negative:

• Negative is when, considering the hydration status of the patient before the treatment (O), the difference between the achieved patient fluid removal at a certain point in treatment (A) and the prescribed/set fluid removal until that moment (B) is negative (AO − BO < 0). A negative fluid balance error means the treatment removed less fluid than expected and, depending on the magnitude of the volume error, it can be a source of patient volume expansion.

• Positive is when, considering the hydration status of the patient before the treatment (O), the difference between the achieved patient fluid removal at a certain point in treatment (C) and the prescribed/set fluid removal until that moment (B) is positive (CO − BO > 0). A positive fluid balance error means the treatment removed more fluid than expected and, depending on the magnitude of the volume error, it can be source of patient volume contraction.

Extracorporeal Therapies and Treatments

Extracorporeal treatments can be categorized according to session frequency and duration.

Continuous Therapies

CRRTs have been identified as the most appropriate modality for the management of hemodynamically unstable patients with AKI. This notwithstanding, the intense effort required to perform CRRT, including the need for specialized expertise and specific equipment, the necessity of continuous anticoagulation, the nursing workload, continuous alarm vigilance, and its higher cost, make this therapy still imperfect. CRRT can be provided in various forms depending on resources, patient needs, and staff skills (Figure 3.1).

CRRT is any extracorporeal blood purification therapy that aims to substitute kidney function over an extended period of time. It ensures better hemodynamic stability, lesser transcellular solute shifts, and better tolerance

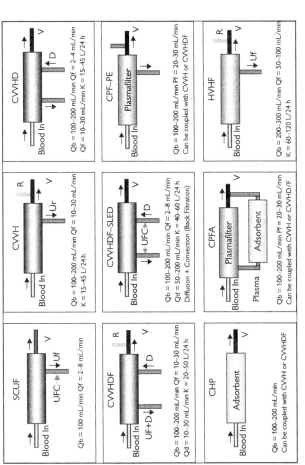

Figure 3.1 Continuous extracorporeal therapies and treatments.

to fluid removal than intermittent extracorporeal modalities. Prescription is usually reviewed every 24 hour or less, depending on patient needs, and it can respond very well to the continuously changing needs of the critically ill patient.

Nowadays, CRRT treatments are performed using a double-lumen catheter as vascular access, a venovenous technique whereby blood is driven by a pump through a filter via an extracorporeal circuit, originating from a vein and returning to the same vein. In the past (until the late 1980s), these therapies were commonly performed by applying an arterio-venous extracorporeal circuit. This modality has fallen into disuse and is not discussed further.

Slow, Continuous Ultrafiltration

Slow, continuous ultrafiltration is a therapy based on the slow removal of plasma water only. It is performed to manage patients with pathological and refractory fluid overload, with or without renal dysfunction. Its primary aim is to achieve safe and effective correction of fluid overload. It is not suitable to achieve clearance of solutes.

Continuous Venovenous Hemofiltration

Continuous venovenous hemofiltration is a form of continuous hemofiltration. The mechanism of transmembrane solute transport is convection. Ultrafiltrate is replaced partially or completely with appropriate replacement fluids to achieve solute clearance and volume control. Replacement fluid can be infused before (predilution) and/or after (postdilution) the hemofilter.

Continuous Venovenous Hemodialysis

Continuous venovenous hemodialysis (CVVHD) is a form of continuous HD characterized by slow countercurrent/co-current dialysate flow into the dialysate compartment of the hemodialyzer. The main mechanism of transmembrane solute transport is diffusion.

Continuous Venovenous Hemodiafiltration

Continuous venovenous hemodiafiltration combines hemodialysis and hemofiltration modalities. Ultrafiltrate is replaced partially or completely by replacement fluid (pre- or post-infusion), and countercurrent/co-current dialysate flows into the dialysate compartment. Solute clearance is achieved via diffusive and convective clearances. Both small- and large-molecular weight solutes are removed.

Continuous Venovenous High-Flux Hemodialysis

Continuous venovenous high-flux hemodialysis consists of the same treatment as CVVHD, but is carried out using high-flux membranes. Because of the high-flux properties of the membrane, a convective component of solute clearance is achieved even if replacement fluid is not infused.

Intermittent Therapies

Intermittent therapies involve techniques carried out in sessions of 3 to 5 hours. Intermittent techniques require adequate vascular access, specifically trained nurses, and a specific water processing and sterilization procedure that produces pure water for dialysate. Because the treatment time is relatively short, blood purification efficiency needs to be greater than that of CRRT. The most commonly prescribed intermittent therapies are intermittent hemodialysis, intermittent hemofiltration, intermittent hemodiafiltration, and intermittent high-flux dialysis. Many other therapies are available that combine different modalities, but because these are not usually performed in the ICU, they are not discussed in this chapter.

Hybrid Therapies

Hybrid therapies are so called because they share characteristics of both intermittent and continuous techniques in terms of frequency and duration. These therapies attempt to optimize the pros and cons of both modalities: efficient solute removal, slower ultrafiltration rates for hemodynamic stability, less anticoagulant exposure, lesser time and costs, decreased nurse workload, and improved ICU workflow. Hybrid therapies encompass various specific "discontinuous" RRT modalities: sustained low-efficiency dialysis, slow low-efficiency extended daily dialysis, prolonged intermittent daily renal replacement therapy, extended daily dialysis, extended daily dialysis with filtration, extended dialysis, go-slow dialysis, and accelerated venovenous hemofiltration.

Hybrid therapies are usually performed with standard intermittent hemodialysis equipment, including machines, filters, extracorporeal blood circuits, and online fluid production for dialysate and ultrafiltrate infusion. Solute removal is largely diffusive, but variants with a convective component, such as slow low-efficiency extended daily dialysis with filtration (SLED-f) and accelerated venovenous hemofiltration, are possible.

The most commonly prescribed hybrid therapy is sustained low-efficiency dialysis. It is a technique that uses reduced blood and dialysate flows and is usually limited to 10 to 12 hours. There are limited data on the application of these techniques in appropriately powered studies

Other Extracorporeal Treatments

An important section of blood purification techniques performed in the ICU involves other so-called extracorporeal treatments. Mainly derived from RRT, these treatments are usually performed to clear toxins and solutes generally not removable by "classic" RRT, or to support single- or multiple-organ dysfunctions.

Therapeutic Plasma Exchange

Therapeutic plasma exchange (TPE) consists of the automated removal of plasma (plasmapheresis) and its replacement (exchange) with a suitable fluid composed of fresh frozen plasma and albumin in a ratio usually of 2:1. TPE is performed through a centrifugal-based system or a very high-permeable membrane-based filtration that separates plasma from cellular elements of blood. In membrane-based TPE, pore sizes ranging between 0.2 μm and 0.6 μm allow a sieving coefficient of 0.9 to 1.0 for molecules with a molecular weight greater than 500 kDa.

Continuous plasma exchange is a therapy derived from TPE that is performed with lower flow rates and for a longer period of time. Usually, large quantities of plasma substitute infusion are required. Single or repeated sessions can be performed as pure continuous plasma exchange or in conjunction with other purification techniques.

A particular type of TPE is therapeutic plasma exchange with selected reinfusion, in which the rate of infusion of fresh frozen plasma and albumin can be reduced dramatically. In particular, the plasma is first separated in a plasma filter and then flows into a standard filter (cutoff, 35 kDa) from which the effluent, depurated of high-molecular weight solutes, is reinfused into the main circuit.

Treatment Evaluation Methods: The "Dose" in RRT

During the past decades, increasing attention has been paid to the quantification of the delivered "dose" of RRT. Although the most appropriate dose has not been established for the majority of clinical conditions, large studies have demonstrated a direct relationship between dose and survival, both for intermittent and for continuous RRT. On the basis of those studies, the appropriate prescribed dose of continuous RRT has recently been standardized at 20 to 25 mL/kg per hour. However, application to clinical practice still needs to be improved.

New evidence has shown that fluid balance may be as important as blood purification in critically ill patients with renal dysfunction. It has become increasingly clear that the magnitude of fluid removal and the use of RRT to optimize fluid status should become part of the "dose" calculation.

Studies in special settings, such as septic RRT, pediatric RRT, and RRT during extracorporeal membrane oxygenation, have recently shown important results. New applications in clinical practice have demonstrated the important consequences of technical improvement in the current and future care of these patients.

Dose identifies the amount of blood cleared of waste products and toxins by the extracorporeal circuit. Operatively, dose is measured as the removal rate of a representative solute. Urea, usually considered a uremic toxin marker, is used most often to quantify dose because it is an indicator of protein catabolism and is retained in kidney failure. However, urea metabolism and concentration do not measure the metabolism of all the accumulated solutes in renal failure, because different solutes differ in their kinetic parameters and volume of distribution.

Originally, this solute-based approach was developed to measure the dose of dialysis prescribed to patients with end-stage renal disease. In those patients, the application of this approach is relatively simple and correlates well with patient outcome. However, when using CRRT to treat critically ill patients, other measures of adequacy and dose should be considered, including measurement of flows across the dialysis machine, which could be an easier and more reproducible means to estimate dose.

Efficiency

Identified as a clearance (K), the efficiency represents the volume of blood cleared of a solute for a given period of time. It can be expressed as the ratio of blood volume over time (e.g., milliliters per minute, milliliters per hour, liters per hour, liters per 24 hours) and is generally normalized to ideal patient weight (milliliters per kilogram per hour). Efficiency depends on the reference molecules chosen (molecular size), removal mechanisms (diffusion, convection, or both), and circuit operational characteristics (e.g., flows, types of filters). Efficiency can be used to compare different RRT treatments applied with the same modality (e.g., continuous venovenous hemofiltration, CVVHD, continuous venovenous hemodiafiltration) using different settings and operational characteristics.

Intensity

Intensity can be defined by Efficiency × Time. Operatively, intensity represents the blood volume cleared of a solute for a certain period of time. It can be expressed as milliliters or liters per unit time (minute, hours, or a whole day). When comparing RRT modalities with different duration times, the use of intensity is more appropriate than the use of efficiency. For example, despite its low efficiency, the use of CRRT for a long period of time results in increased treatment intensity.

Efficacy

Efficacy measures the effective removal of a specific solute resulting from a given treatment in a given patient. It can be identified as the ratio of the entire volume cleared during the treatment to the volume of distribution of that solute. Operatively, efficacy is a dimensionless number and it can be defined numerically as the ratio between intensity and the volume of distribution of a specific solute.

Urea is the usual marker to describe the kinetics of the small molecules retained during renal failure. Because it readily traverses cell membranes, its volume of distribution is equal to the entire body water.

Conclusions

When faced with a complex patient, practitioners can use a growing variety of extracorporeal treatment options. Although definitive evidence is still lacking in many areas, there is worldwide consensus that the degree of hemodynamic stability is the main determinant of the choice of RRT modality, as shown in two large studies on the appropriate dose of dialysis. Understanding the importance of dose quantification—and ensuring the delivery of an adequate dose—are critical determinants of patient outcome. Although preliminary evidence suggests that timely initiation of RRT is important, definitive studies to address this issue are currently in progress. For patients with multiple-organ failure, an increasingly rich panoply of options is being developed, including extracorporeal treatments for sepsis, and cardiac, pulmonary, and liver failure.

Understanding the basic mechanisms and the practical applications underlying the process of RRT is essential to implement adequate treatment choices to the individual patient. Although apparently simple, these choices are in reality complex, and specific to each clinical situation. Terminologies and nomenclatures that are solid and shared worldwide will contribute to a thorough understanding of the basics and the correct application of such technologies, and add to future developments in the field.

Key References

Cerda J, Ronco C. Choosing a renal replacement therapy in acute kidney injury: technical and clinical considerations. In: Kellum JA, Cerda J, eds. *Renal and Metabolic Disorders*. Pittsburgh: Oxford University Press; 2013: 77–90.

Cerda J, Ronco C. Modalities of continuous renal replacement therapy: technical and clinical considerations. *Semin Dial*. 2009;22(2):114–122.

Cruz D, Bobek I, Lentini P, Soni S, Chionh CY, Ronco C. Machines for continuous renal replacement therapy. *Semin Dial*. 2009;22(2):123–132.

KDIGO clinical practice guideline for acute kidney injury. *Kidney Int*. 2012;2(suppl):1–138.

Tolwani A. Continuous renal replacement therapy for acute kidney injury. *N Engl J Med*. 2012;367(26):2505–2514.

Chapter 4

Basic Principles of Solute Transport

Zhongping Huang, Jeffrey J. Letteri, Claudio Ronco, and William R. Clark

Characterization of Filter Performance in Continuous Renal Replacement Therapy

Several different parameters can be used to characterize filter performance in continuous renal replacement therapy (CRRT). Two of the most common parameters, clearance and sieving coefficient, are discussed here.

Clearance

Quantification of dialytic solute removal is complicated by the confusion relating to the relationship between clearance and mass removal for different therapies. By definition, solute clearance (K) is the ratio of mass removal rate (N) to blood solute concentration (C_B):

$$K = \frac{N}{C_B}.$$

[4.1]

From a kinetic perspective, Figure 4.1 depicts the relevant flows for determining continuous renal replacement therapy (CRRT) clearances whereas Figure 4.2 provides the solute clearance expressions, which differ from those used in conventional hemodialysis. In the latter therapy, the mass removal rate (i.e., the rate at which the hemodialyzer extracts solute from blood into the dialysate) is estimated by measuring the difference in solute concentration between the arterial and venous lines. In other words, a "blood-side" clearance approach is used. On the other hand, in CRRT, the mass removal rate is estimated by measuring the actual amount of solute appearing in the effluent. The mass removal rate is the product of the effluent flow rate (Q_{EFF}) and the effluent concentration of the solute (C_{EFF}). In continuous venovenous hemodialysis and continuous venovenous hemodiafiltration (CVVHDF), the effluent is dialysate and diafiltrate, respectively. For these therapies, the extent of solute extraction from the blood is estimated by the

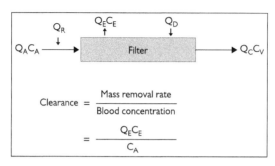

Figure 4.1 Relevant flow and concentration considerations for the determination of solute clearance in continuous renal replacement therapy. The modality represented is continuous venovenous hemodiafiltration. Q_A: arterial blood flow rate; Q_V: venous blood flow rate; Q_E: effluent flow rate; Q_D: dialysate flow rate; Q_R: replacement fluid rate; C_A: arterial blood solute concentration; C_V: venous blood solute concentration; C_E: effluent solute concentration;

equilibration ratio (E), also known as the *degree of effluent saturation*. The benchmark for efficiency in these therapies is the volume of fluid (dialysate and/or replacement fluid) required to achieve a certain solute clearance target (discussed later).

Clearance in postdilution continuous venovenous hemofiltration (CVVH) is the product of the sieving coefficient (discussed in the next section) and the ultrafiltration rate (Q_{UF}). For small solutes like urea and creatinine, the sieving coefficient is, essentially, one (under normal hemofilter operation). Therefore, small solute clearance in postdilution CVVH is, essentially, equal to the Q_{UF}. On the other hand, estimation of clearance in predilution CVVH has to account for the fact that the blood solute concentrations are reduced by dilution of the blood before it enters the hemofilter. Thus, the clearance has a "dilution factor," which is represented by the third term on the right

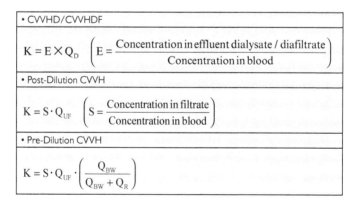

Figure 4.2 Solute Clearance in CRRT

side of Eq. [4.1]. This term essentially is the ratio of the blood flow rate (Q_B) to the sum of Q_B and the replacement fluid rate reinfused upstream of the hemofilter (Q_R^{PRE}). (The actual blood flow parameter, Q_{BW}, is blood water flow rate.) In essence, the dilution factor can be viewed as a measure of the extent to which predilution differs from postdilution for a specific combination of Q_B and Q_{UF}.

Sieving Coefficient

When a filter is operated as a hemofilter (i.e., ultrafiltration with no dialysate flow, such as CVVH), solute mass transfer occurs almost exclusively by convection. Convective solute removal is determined primarily by membrane pore size and treatment ultrafiltration rate. Mean pore size is the major determinant of a hemofilter's ability to prevent or allow the transport of a specific solute. The sieving coefficient (SC) represents the degree to which a particular membrane permits the passage of a specific solute:

$$SC = \frac{C_{UF}}{C_P}. \qquad [4.2]$$

In this equation, C_{UF} and C_P are the solute concentrations in the ultrafiltrate and the plasma (water), respectively.

Regardless of membrane type, all hemofilters in the "virgin" state have small solute SC values of one, and these values are typically not reported by manufacturers. SC values for solutes of larger molecular weight are more applicable, and manufacturers frequently provide data for one or more middle-molecule surrogates, such as vitamin B_{12}, inulin, cytochrome C, and myoglobin. As is the case for solute clearance, the relationship between the SC and solute molecular weight is highly dependent on membrane mean pore size.

SC data provided by manufacturers are usually derived from in vitro experimental systems in which (nonprotein-containing) aqueous solutions are used as the blood compartment fluid. In actual clinical practice, nonspecific adsorption of plasma proteins to a filter membrane effectively reduces the permeability of the membrane. Consequently, in vivo SC values are typically less than those derived from aqueous experiments, sometimes by a considerable amount.

Transmembrane Solute Removal Mechanisms

The most common way in which solute removal occurs during CRRT is passage across the filter membrane into the effluent. Based on the specific CRRT modality used, diffusion, convection, or a combination of these two mechanisms are operative. Figure 4.3

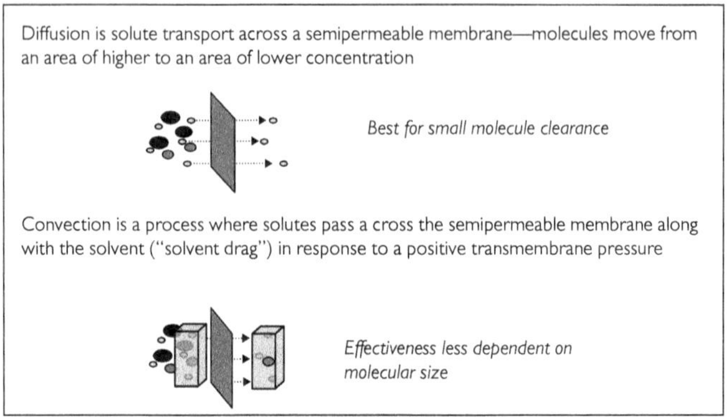

Diffusion is solute transport across a semipermeable membrane—molecules move from an area of higher to an area of lower concentration

Best for small molecule clearance

Convection is a process where solutes pass a cross the semipermeable membrane along with the solvent ("solvent drag") in response to a positive transmembrane pressure

Effectiveness less dependent on molecular size

Figure 4.3 Mechanisms of diffusion and convection.

Diffusion

Diffusion is the process of transport in which molecules that are present in a solvent and can cross a semipermeable membrane freely tend to move from the region of higher concentration to the region of lower concentration. In reality, molecules present a random movement. However, because they tend to reach the same concentration in the available space occupied by the solvent, the number of particles crossing the membrane toward the region of lower concentration is greater statistically. Therefore, this transport mechanism occurs in the presence of a concentration gradient for solutes that are not restricted in diffusion by the porosity of the membrane. In addition to a transmembrane concentration gradient, Fick's Law states diffusive solute is influenced by the following:

• Membrane characteristics: surface area, thickness, porosity
• Solute diffusion coefficient (primarily a function of molecular weight)
• Solution temperature

Based on the previous discussion, the clearance of a given solute can be predicted with reasonable certainty under a given set of operating conditions. However, several factors may lead to a divergence between theoretical and empirically derived values. As an example, protein binding or electrical charges in the solute may affect the final clearance value negatively. Conversely, convection may result in a measured clearance value that is significantly greater than the value based on a "pure" diffusion assumption. Diffusion is an efficient transport mechanism for the removal of relatively small solutes; but, as solute molecular weight increases, diffusion becomes limited and the relative importance of convection increases.

Convection

Convection is the mass transfer mechanism associated with ultrafiltration of plasma water. If a solute is small enough to pass through the pore structure of the membrane, it is driven ("dragged") across the membrane in association with the ultrafiltered plasma water. This movement of plasma water is a consequence of a transmembrane pressure (TMP) gradient. Quantitatively, the ultrafiltration flux (J_F), defined as the ultrafiltration rate normalized to membrane surface area, can be described by

$$J_F = L_h \times TMP. \qquad [4.3]$$

In this equation, L_h is the membrane-specific hydraulic permeability (measured in milliliters per hour per millimeters mercury per meters squared), and TMP is a function of both the hydrostatic and oncotic pressure gradients.

The related convective flux of a given solute is a function mainly of the following parameters:

- Ultrafiltration rate
- Blood solute concentration
- Membrane sieving properties

In clinical practice, however, because plasma proteins and other factors modify the "native" properties of the membrane, the final observed sieving coefficient is less than that expected from a simple theoretical calculation. As noted earlier, nonspecific adsorption of plasma proteins (i.e., secondary membrane formation) occurs instantaneously to an extracorporeal membrane after exposure to blood. This changes the effective permeability of the membrane and can be explained by the action of proteins essentially to "plug" or block a certain percentage of membrane pores. Postdilution fluid replacement tends to accentuate secondary membrane effects because protein concentrations are increased within the membrane fibers (resulting from hemoconcentration). On the other hand, greater blood flow rates work to attenuate this process because the shear effect created by the blood disrupts the binding of proteins to the membrane surface

Kinetic Considerations for Different CRRT Techniques

In CVVH, high-flux membranes are used and the prevalent mechanism of solute transport is convection. Ultrafiltration rates in excess of the amount required for volume control are prescribed, requiring partial or total replacement of ultrafiltrate losses with reinfusion (replacement) fluid. Replacement fluid can either be infused before the hemofilter (predilution) or after the hemofilter (postdilution). Postdilution hemofiltration is limited inherently by the attainable blood flow rate and the associated filtration fraction constraint.

On the other hand, from a mass transfer perspective, the use of predilution has several potential advantages over postdilution. First, both hematocrit and blood total protein concentration are reduced significantly before the entry of blood into the hemofilter. This effective reduction in the red cell and protein content of the blood attenuates the secondary membrane and concentration polarization phenomena described earlier, resulting in improved mass transfer. Predilution also affects mass transfer favorably as a result of augmented flow in the blood compartment because prefilter mixing of blood and replacement fluid occurs. This process achieves a relatively high membrane shear rate, which also reduces solute–membrane interactions. Last, predilution may also enhance mass transfer for some compounds by creating concentration gradients that induce solute movement out of red blood cells.

However, the major drawback of predilution hemofiltration is its relatively low efficiency, resulting in relatively high replacement fluid requirements to achieve a given solute clearance. In a group of patients treated with a "traditional" blood flow rate for CRRT, the efficiency loss associated with predilution has been quantified. Troyanov and colleagues demonstrated the significant negative effect on efficiency when a relatively low Q_B (<150 mL/min) is used with a relatively high Q_{UF} and Q_R in predilution CVVH. This specific combination of Q_B = 125–150 mL/min and Q_{UF} = 4.5 L/h (75 mL/min) is associated with a loss of efficiency of 30% to 40% relative to postdilution for several different solutes. In other words, to achieve the same solute clearance, 30% to 40% more replacement fluid is required in predilution under these conditions, relative to postdilution under the same conditions. However, it should be noted the likelihood of achieving such an ultrafiltration rate in postdilution is very remote at such a low blood flow rate, because this requires a filtration fraction in excess of 50%. This condition is likely to lead to very short-term filter patency.

In CVVHDF, a high-flux hemodiafilter is used and the operating principles of hemodialysis and hemofiltration are combined. As such, this therapy may allow for an optimal combination of diffusion and convection to provide clearances for a very broad range of solutes. Dialysate is circulated in countercurrent mode to blood and, at the same time, ultrafiltration is obtained in excess of the desired fluid loss from the patient. The ultrafiltrate is replaced with replacement fluid partially or totally, either in predilution or postdilution mode. Later generation CRRT machines allow a combination of predilution and postdilution with the aim of combining the advantages of both reinfusion techniques. Information from the chronic hemodiafiltration literature suggests a combination of predilution and postdilution may be optimal in terms of clearance and operational parameters. This may also be the case for CVVHDF in acute kidney injury (AKI), although this possibility has not been assessed carefully. The optimal balance is most likely dictated by the specific set of CVVHDF operating conditions—namely, blood flow rate, dialysate flow rate, ultrafiltration rate, and hemodiafilter type.

Because of the markedly lower flow rates used and clearances obtained in CVVHDF, the effect of simultaneous diffusion and convection on overall solute removal is quite different from the situation in chronic hemodiafiltration. In the latter application, diffusion and convection interact in such a manner that total solute removal is significantly less than what is expected if the individual components are simply added together. On the other hand, in CVVHDF, the small solute concentration gradient along the axial length of the hemodiafilter (i.e., extraction) is minimal compared with what is seen in chronic hemodiafiltration, in which extraction ratios of 50% or more are the norm. Thus, the minimal diffusion-related change in small solute concentrations along the hemodiafilter length allows any additional clearance related to convection to be simply additive to the diffusive component

Troyanov and coworkers have performed a direct clinical comparison of CVVHDF and predilution CVVH with respect to urea and β2-microglobulin (B2M) clearance at a "traditional" blood flow rate of 125 mL/min. The study compared clearances at the same effluent rate over an effluent range of up to 4.5 L/h. As Figure 4.4 indicates, urea clearance was greater in CVVHDF than in predilution CVVH and, in fact, the difference between the two therapies increased as effluent rate increased. These results are consistent with the "penalizing" effect of predilution, which is especially pronounced at low blood

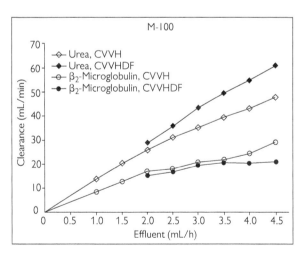

Figure 4.4 Comparison of solute clearance in predilution continuous venovenous hemofiltration and continuous venovenous hemodiafiltration.

Reprinted with permission from (Troyanov S, Cardinal J, Geadah D, Parent D, Courteau S, Caron S, Leblanc M: Solute clearances during continuous venovenous haemofiltration at various ultrafiltration flow rates using Multiflow-100 and HF1000 filters. Nephrol Dial Transplant 2003;18:961–966).

flow rates. For B2M, the results are contrary to the "conventional wisdom," which would suggest a purely convective therapy such as CVVH should be inherently superior to a partly convective therapy like CVVHDF for clearance of a molecule this size. However, once again, the penalty of predilution in CVVH is apparent, as the B2M clearances for the two modalities are equivalent, except at very high effluent rates (>3.5 L/h). Until the effect of greater blood flow rates on solute clearances in CRRT can be assessed, these and other data suggest CVVHDF is a logical modality choice to achieve the broadest spectrum of solute molecular weight range in the most efficient way.

Conclusion

Rational prescription of CRRT to critically ill patients with AKI is predicated on an understanding of the basic principles of solute and water removal. In this chapter, the major ways in which filter function is characterized clinically have been reviewed. In addition, the fundamental mechanisms for solute and fluid transport have been discussed. Last, these principles have been applied in a therapeutic context to the various CRRT modalities used by clinicians managing patients with AKI.

Key References

Brunet S, Leblanc M, Geadah D, Parent D, Courteau S, Cardinal J. Diffusive and convective solute clearances during continuous renal replacement therapy at various dialysate and ultrafiltration flow rates. *Am J Kidney Dis*. 1999;34:486–492.

Clark WR, Turk JE, Kraus MA, Gao D. Dose determinants in continuous renal replacement therapy. *Artif Organs*. 2003;27:815–820.

Henderson LW. Biophysics of ultrafiltration and hemofiltration. In: Jacobs C, ed. *Replacement of Renal Function by Dialysis*. 4th ed. Dordrecht: Kluwer Academic Publishers; 1996:114–118.

Huang Z, Letteri JJ, Clark WR, Ronco C. Operational characteristics of continuous renal replacement therapy modalities used for critically ill patients with acute kidney injury. *Int J Artif Organs*. 2008;31:525–534.

Huang Z, Letteri JJ, Clark WR, Zhang W, Gao D, Ronco C. Ultrafiltration rate as dose surrogate in pre-dilution hemofiltration. *Int J Artif Organs*. 2007;30:124–132.

Troyanov S, Cardinal J, Geadah D, et al. Solute clearances during continuous venovenous haemofiltration at various ultrafiltration flow rates using Multiflow-100 and HF1000 filters. *Nephrol Dial Transplant*. 2003;18:961–966.

Chapter 5

Principles of Fluid Management in the Intensive Care Unit

Rinaldo Bellomo and Sean M. Bagshaw

Approach to Fluid Balance during Continuous Renal Replacement Therapy

The prescription of continuous renal replacement therapy (CRRT)-related fluid management and its integration into overall patient fluid management can be assisted by a specific order chart (Table 5.1) for the machine fluid balance.

The chart indicates to the nurse how to set the machine and how to achieve the planned hourly fluid balance. However, in the intensive care unit, the fluid needs of the patients are not static and require frequent review. Patients often receive large volumes of obligatory oral and intravenous fluids daily that also need to be accounted for when making fluid balance calculations. For example, should the same patient require the administration of 600 mL fresh frozen plasma over 2 hours before an invasive procedure, necessary adjustments to the order should be made with specification for the duration of change and the reasons (Table 5.2).

The fluid balance prescription related to the machine can be related usefully to the patient, and a fluid balance prescription describing the overall patient fluid balance goal for a 12-hour time period is useful for the purpose of informing the nurse of the broad goals of fluid therapy for a given patient. These goals may be expressed in an additional prescription attached to the previous machine fluid balance chart (Table 5.3).

Practical Considerations

The goals can be achieved by means of physician and nursing education, and by ensuring that no CRRT session is started unless such orders are written clearly and legibly, and signed and accompanied by the physician's printed name and contact number. They also require the regular recording of fluid balance on an hourly basis, and its correct final addition of fluid losses and gains. This

Table 5.1 Example of prescription of machine fluid balance during continuous renal replacement therapy

Technique	Dialysate Flow Rate	Replacement Fluid Flow rate	Effluent Flow Rate	Anticoagulant Infusion Flow Rate	Machine Fluid Balance
Continuous venovenous hemodia-filtration	1000 mL/h	1000 mL/h	2300 mL/hr	100 mL/h	−200 mL/h

documentation can be done in a computerized system or may be added by the nurse at the bedside using a pocket calculator and then charted. This process allows the creation of a running hourly balance, which is useful in ensuring that progress is being made at the appropriate speed, in the appropriate direction, and in the prescribed amount.

Expected Outcomes, Potential Problems, Cautions, and Benefits

The expected outcome of a systematic process for the prescription, delivery, and monitoring of fluids during CRRT is the ability to ensure the patient receives prescribed therapy in a safe and effective manner. This approach minimizes errors and their consequences (persistent fluid overload or dangerous intravascular volume depletion).

Despite this careful approach, problems can still arise. A relatively common problem is related to downtime (time during which CRRT is not operative as a result of filter clotting or a procedure or investigation out of the intensive care unit). Under such circumstances, the prescribed fluid removal cannot proceed as planned. If the patient has 5 hours of downtime, then the consequence may be that close to 1 L of planned fluid removal fails to occur (assuming a fluid balance

Table 5.2 Example of alteration of continuous renal replacement therapy fluid balance prescription

Technique	Dialysate Flow Rate	Replacement Fluid Flow Rate	Effluent Flow Rate	Anticoagulant Infusion Flow Rate	Machine Fluid Balance
Continuous venovenous hemodia-filtration	1000 mL/h	1000 mL/h	2600 mL/h	100 mL/h	−500 mL/h (for 2 hours only during Fresh frozen plasma (FFP) treatment)

Table 5.3 **Example of patient fluid balance prescription**				
Patient	Medical Record No.	Overall Fluid Balance from Midnight to 12:00 Noon	Overall Fluid Balance from 12:00 Noon to 12:00 Midnight	Right Atrial Pressure Notification Range
Name	00123	−1000 mL	−1000 mL/h	<6 or >15 mmHg

of −200 mL/h). Moreover, during this downtime, patients may be administered additional fluid that counters earlier fluid balance goals. If this happens, the physician and the nurse need to be alert to the consequences and respond appropriately. This action may require an adjustment in fluid removal during the ensuing 12 hours or 24 hours that safely compensates for the downtime by increasing the hourly net ultrafiltration rate by, for example, an extra 100 mL/h.

Due consideration needs to be paid to specific patients in whom such fluid removal may be problematic. However, typically, machine net ultrafiltration rates of 300 to 400 mL/h are well tolerated in fluid-overloaded patients. Nonetheless, caution should be exerted and the patient's condition should be reviewed frequently.

Another relatively common problem relates to frequent interruptions of therapy as a result of machine alarms. In some patients who are agitated or who have frequent leg flexion in the presence of a femoral access catheter, or who sit up and move in the bed in the presence of a subclavian access device, the machine pressure alarms may be triggered frequently. In addition, other alarms related to substitution fluids bag or waste bag changes interrupt treatment, which may lead to periods of 5 to 10 minutes in any given hour and, over a day, may create downtime and failure to achieve fluid balance goals. It is often prudent to prescribe a greater fluid loss than desired to compensate for these factors. Most machines allow the operator to check the actual fluid removal achieved over a given time. Such checks should be done to ensure the correct fluid removal is entered into the fluid balance calculations; many nursing protocols mandate a fluid balance check each hour, particularly for inexperienced nurses. Last, during such periods of circuit instability, machine-based fluid errors may also occur and nurses and doctors need to be aware of such possibilities and remain alert to patient hemodynamics.

The benefits of such continuous monitoring of fluid delivery and removal are many. They include frequent patient assessment, vigilance with regard to other simultaneous therapies, attention to detail, avoidance of dangerous swings in fluid status and competent and detailed machine operation.

Summary

Attention to fluid balance during CRRT is of great clinical importance. Inadequate fluid removal leads to clinical complications, especially in relation to weaning from mechanical ventilation. Excessive fluid removal can cause hypovolemia and hypotension, and retards renal recovery. Best practice in this field can only be achieved by a systematic combination of frequent and thoughtful assessment, attention to detail, rigorous and vigilant monitoring of fluid input and output, and clear and explicit descriptions and prescription of the goals of therapy with regard to both machine settings and patient management.

Key References

Bagshaw S, Baldwin I, Fealy N, Bellomo R. Fluid balance error in continuous renal replacement therapy: a technical note. *Int J Artif Organs*. 2007;30:435–440.

Bagshaw S, Bellomo R. Fluid resuscitation and the septic kidney. *Curr Opin Crit Care*. 2006;12:527–530.

Bagshaw SM, Bellomo R. The influence of volume management on outcome. *Curr Opin Crit Care*. 2007;13:541–548.

Bagshaw SM, Brophy PD, Cruz D, Ronco C. Fluid balance as a biomarker: impact of fluid overload on outcome in critically ill patients with acute kidney injury. *Crit Care*. 2008;12:169.

Prowle JR, Bellomo R. Fluid administration and the kidney. *Curr Opin Crit Care*. 2013;19:308–314.

Chapter 6

Indications, Timing, and Patient Selection

John A. Kellum, Raghavan Murugan, and Mitra K. Nadim

Indications for Renal Replacement Therapy

Indications for renal replacement therapy (RRT) fall into two broad categories: so-called "renal" (i.e., to address the consequences of renal failure specifically) and "nonrenal" (without necessitating renal failure). Although the distinction is not always precise, it is a reasonably easy way to categorize indications for RRT.

Renal Indications

The manifestations of acute kidney injury (AKI), as discussed in Chapter 1 and summarized in Table 6.1, include oliguria, (which leads to fluid overload), azotemia (which leads to a host of clinical complications), hyperkalemia, and metabolic acidosis. Although there is no consensus regarding the precise level of dysfunction in any of these areas that should prompt initiation of RRT, general agreement exists on the following general indications for RRT:

- Fluid overload (e.g., pulmonary edema)
- Oliguria or anuria (urine output of <0.3 mL/kg/h for ≥24 hours or anuria for ≥12 hours)
- Azotemia with uremic symptoms
- Hyperkalemia associated with electrocardiographic changes
- Severe acidosis

Fluid Overload

Multiple studies show that fluid overload is associated independently with mortality. Fluid overload usually occurs in the setting of oliguria, but it may occur simply because urine output is insufficient to maintain fluid balance in the face of large volume input, even if oliguria is not present. Although an initial

Table 6.1 Manifestations of acute kidney injury

System	Complication	Mechanism	Clinical features
Cardiovascular	Fluid overload	Salt/water retention	Edema, heart failure, hypertension
Electrolyte and acid–base	Hyponatremia, hyperkalemia, acidosis, azotemia	Impaired free water excretion, chloride accumulation	Hypotension, impaired glucose metabolism, decreased muscle protein synthesis, cardiac dysrhythmias
Gastrointestinal	Impaired nutrient absorption, gastrointestinal bleeding, abdominal compartment syndrome	Bowel edema, fluid overload	Nausea, vomiting, decreased mucosal/ intestinal absorption, increased intra-abdominal pressures
Hematological	Anemia, platelet dysfunction	Decreased erythropoietin, decreased von Willebrand factor	Anemia, bleeding
Immune	Infections, immune suppression	Impaired neutrophil function	Nosocomial infections, severe sepsis
Nervous	Encephalopathy	Uremic toxins, hyponatremia	Asterixis, delirium, stupor, coma
Respiratory	Pleural effusions, pulmonary edema	Fluid overload, decreased oncotic pressure, ?direct uremic toxicity	Pleural effusion, pulmonary edema, respiratory failure

trial of pharmacological treatment to induce diuresis may serve as a temporizing measure, patients with symptomatic fluid overload (e.g., worsening oxygenation) in addition to severe AKI characterized by concomitant indications for RRT initiation (i.e., hyperkalemia, uremia) or those with life-threatening complications of fluid overload should be treated urgently with RRT.

Although most clinicians will attempt diuretics before initiation of RRT, there is a wide variation with regard to how long or intense such a trial should be or how the success is defined. Obviously, it is desirable to avoid RRT, however there is little evidence to suggest that diuretics can be successful in achieving this goal.

More important, attempts to increase urine output with diuretics should only be directed toward treatment of fluid overload or hyperkalemia, not oliguria per se. The Acute Dialysis Quality Initiative addressed the indications for mechanical fluid removal in 2012. Mechanical fluid removal should be considered under the following circumstances: (1) when fluid overload is established and after diuretic therapy is ineffective or has failed; (2) in patients with life-threatening fluid overload and significantly reduced renal function (e.g., low glomerular filtration rate [GFR]) or poor renal perfusion (e.g., cardiogenic shock) in whom diuretic therapy is *likely* to fail; (3) in patients at high risk of fluid accumulation (e.g., need for massive blood products, parenteral nutrition, or high-volume drug infusion), who should be started on ultrafiltration to prevent fluid overload, (4) if complications associated with use of diuretics, such as hyponatremia, severe metabolic alkalosis, hypomagnesemia, severe hypokalemia and worsening kidney function, are present; and (5) in patients in whom fluid overload occurs in the context of severe acute or chronic kidney disease and uremic symptoms.

Diuretic Therapy

A loop diuretic such as furosemide is given in a dose of 20 to 40 mg intravenously (IV) (Table 6.2). If this dose is ineffective, a higher dose can be tried within 30 to 60 minutes. Higher doses may be needed if the patient has previously received diuretic therapy (Table 6.1). If bolus doses of 80 mg every 6 hours are ineffective, an infusion may be started (1–5 mg/h IV). A thiazide diuretic such as chlorothiazide (250–500 mg IV) or metolazone (10–20 mg by mouth) can be used in conjunction with a loop diuretic to improve diuresis. In general, there is no point in continuing diuretic therapy if it is not effective; loop diuretics in particular may be nephrotoxic All diuretics are usually discontinued before initiating RRT.

Azotemia

Azotemia, the retention of urea and other nitrogenous waste products, results from a reduction in GFR and is a cardinal feature of renal failure. However, like oliguria, azotemia represents not only disease, but also a normal response of the kidney to extracellular volume depletion or a decreased renal blood flow. Conversely, a "normal" GFR in the face of volume depletion could be viewed only as renal dysfunction. Thus, changes in urine output and GFR are neither necessary nor sufficient for the diagnosis of renal pathology. Yet, no simple alternative for the diagnosis currently exists.

Azotemia is also a biochemical marker of uremic syndrome, a condition caused by a diverse group of toxins that are excreted normally but build up in the circulation and in the tissues during renal failure. The clinical manifestations of uremic syndrome are shown in Table 6.1.

Although uremic symptoms correlate with the level of urea in the blood, the relationship between blood urea nitrogen (BUN) and uremic symptoms is not

Table 6.2 Diuretic dosing			
Drug	**Oral**	**Intravenous**	**Infusion**
Metolazone	10–20 mg daily		
Chlorothiazide		250–500 mg	
Furosemide	20–40 mg 6–24 hourly	5–80 mg 6–24-hourly	1–10 mg/h
Torsemide	5–20 mg 6–24 hourly	5–20 mg 6–24-hourly	1–5 mg/h
Bumetanide	0.5–1 mg 6–24 hourly	0.5–2 mg 6–24-hourly	1–5 mg/h

consistent across individuals or even within a given individual at different times. Thus, there is no threshold level of BUN that defines uremia or provides a specific indication for RRT. Instead, the provision of RRT and, indeed, decisions regarding timing and intensity should be individualized to patients on the basis of clinical factors and not solely on the basis of biochemical markers.

Hyperkalemia

Hyperkalemia may be severe and can be life-threatening. The risks of hyperkalemia are greatest when it develops rapidly—when serum concentrations in excess of 6 mmol/L may produce cardiac dysrhythmias. The earliest electrocardiographic sign of hyperkalemia is peaking of the T waves. This finding is associated with cardiac irritability and should prompt emergent treatment. Temporary management of severe hyperkalemia (while preparing for RRT) includes intravenous calcium chloride (10 mL of 10% solution) to reduce cardiac irritability and a combination of insulin (10 U IV) and dextrose (50 mL D50) given together over 20 minutes to shift potassium intracellularly (blood glucose should be monitored).

Metabolic Acidosis

Renal failure causes metabolic acidosis by retention of various acid anions (e.g., phosphate, sulfate), as well as from renal tubular dysfunction resulting in hyperchloremic acidosis. Clinical manifestations range from acute alterations in inflammatory cell function to chronic changes in bone mineralization. Mild alterations can be managed using oral sodium bicarbonate or calcium carbonate. RRT is effective in removing acids as well as correcting plasma sodium and chloride balance, and is generally targeted at maintaining an arterial pH of more than 7.30.

"Nonrenal" Indications

So-called nonrenal indications for RRT are to remove various dialyzable substances from the blood. These substances include drugs, poisons, contrast agents, and cytokines.

Drug and Toxin Removal

Blood purification techniques have long been used for removal of various dialyzable drugs and toxins. A list of common drugs and toxins that can be removed readily using RRT is shown in Table 6.3. The majority of poisoning cases do not require treatment with RRT. Indeed, the drugs or toxins that are most commonly responsible for poisoning-related fatalities are not amenable to RRT (e.g., acetaminophen, tricyclic antidepressants, short-acting barbiturates, stimulants, and "street drugs"). In general, the size of the molecule and the degree of protein binding determines the degree to which the substance can be removed (smaller, nonprotein bound substances are easiest to remove). Continuous renal replacement therapy (CRRT) may be effective in

Table 6.3 Common poisonings treated with renal replacement therapy

Substance	Extracorporeal Method	Comments
Methanol	Hemodialysis	RRT should be continued until the serum methanol concentration is less than 25 mg/dL and the anion-gap metabolic acidosis and osmolar gap are normal. Rebound may occur up to 36 hours.
Isopropanol	Hemodialysis	RRT effectively removes isopropanol and acetone, although it is usually unnecessary except in severe cases (prolonged coma, myocardial depression, renal failure).
Ethylene glycol	Hemodialysis	RRT should be continued until the ethylene glycol level is less than 20 mg/dL and metabolic acidosis or other signs of systemic toxicity have been resolved. Rebound may occur up to 24 hours.
Lithium	IHD/CRRT	IHD removes lithium faster, but rebound is a significant problem and can be addressed effectively with CRRT.
Salicylate	IHD/CRRT	Both IHD/CRRT have been reported in the management of salicylate poisoning.
Theophylline	IHD/CRRT/ hemoperfusion	RRT should be continued until clinical improvement and a plasma level less than 20 mg/L is obtained. Rebound may occur.
Valproic acid	IHD/CRRT/ hemoperfusion	At supratherapeutic drug levels, plasma proteins become saturated, and the fraction of unbound drug increases substantially and becomes dialyzable.
Direct thrombin inhibitors (e.g., Dabigatran)	Hemodialysis	Removal of approximately half of the circulating drug by hemodialysis.

Note: Other treatments are also required for many of these substances. CRRT, continuous renal replacement therapy; IHD, intermittent hemodialysis; RRT, renal replacement therapy.

removing substances with greater degrees of protein binding and is sometimes used to remove substances with very long plasma half-lives. Techniques such as sorbent hemoperfusion may also be used for this indication and are discussed further in Chapter 23.

The role of CRRT in the management of acute poisonings is not well established. There is relatively less drug clearance per unit of time compared with intermittent hemodialysis (IHD), but CRRT has a distinct advantage in patients who are hemodynamically unstable and who are unable to tolerate the rapid solute and fluid losses associated with IHD or even other techniques, such as hemoperfusion. CRRT may also be effective for the slow, continuous removal of substances with large volumes of distribution or a high degree of tissue binding, or for substances that are prone to a "rebound phenomenon" (e.g., lithium, procainamide, and methotrexate). In such cases, CRRT may even be used as adjuvant therapy with IHD or hemoperfusion.

Contrast Agents

RRT has been used to remove radiocontrast agents for many years, but the purpose of this treatment has changed over time. In the past, ionic, high-osmolar contrast was used for imaging studies, and RRT was often used to remove these substances and to remove fluid in patients with renal failure who were at risk of congestive heart failure from the large osmotic load. These patients could not excrete the contrast and would develop pulmonary edema after contrast administration. In more recent years, nonionic, low-osmolality, or even iso-osmolar agents have been developed, and the risk of pulmonary edema has decreased significantly. However, all radiocontrast agents are nephrotoxic and CRRT is being advocated by some experts to help prevent so-called *contrast nephropathy*. Standard IHD has been shown to remove radiocontrast agents but does not appear to prevent contrast nephropathy. Despite less efficiency in removing contrast, CRRT has been shown to result in less contrast nephropathy, particularly when it has begun before or in conjunction with contrast administration (Table 6.4). However, the effect is controversial and most centers do not offer RRT currently for prevention of contrast nephropathy.

Cytokines

Many endogenous mediators of sepsis can be removed using continuous veno-venous hemofiltration (CVVH) or continuous venovenous hemodiafiltration (CVVHDF) (dialysis is not able to remove these mediators). This observation has prompted many investigators to attempt to use CVVH as an adjunctive therapy in sepsis. Although it remains controversial regarding whether CVVH offers additional benefit in patients with renal failure and sepsis, available evidence does not support a role of CVVH for the removal of cytokines in patients without renal failure. If CVVH is capable of removing cytokines, the effect of standard "renal-dose" CVVH appears to be small. However, some

Table 6.4 Methods to reduce contrast nephropathy			
	Oral	**IV**	**Dosing***
Saline		0.9% (154 mEq/L)	1 mL/kg/h begun 12 hours or 3 mL/ kg/ h begun 1 hour before procedure and 1 mL/kg/h continuing 6 hours after procedure
NaHCO₃ in water		150 mEq/L	1 mL/kg/h begun 12 hours or 3 mL/kg/h begun 1 hour before procedure and 1 mL/kg/h continuing 6 hours after procedure
N-acetylcysteine	1200 mg every 12 hours	1200 mg every 12 hours	Beginning 24 hours before and continuing 24 hours after procedure

*Dosing ranges are provided as a general guide only; none of the agents in the table are approved for this indication.

individuals appear to respond with improved hemodynamics, especially to higher doses of CVVH (see Chapter 8).

Timing of Renal Replacement Therapy

When to Initiate RRT

The simplest answer to the question "When should RRT be started?" would be when the indications discussed earlier are met. Numerous attempts have been made to reach a consensus on timing of RRT. The Acute Dialysis Quality Initiative first addressed this issue in 2000, but was unable to reach consensus beyond stating that a patient is considered to require RRT when he or she has "an acute fall of GFR and has developed, or is at risk of, clinically significant solute imbalance/toxicity or volume overload." In essence this amounts to saying that RRT should begin when a patient has "symptomatic" acute renal failure (ARF). What constitutes symptomatic ARF is a matter of clinical judgment, and how "at risk" is interpreted. Most, but not all, experts advise that RRT should begin *before* clinical complications occur, but it is often difficult to know exactly when such a point occurs. For example, subtle abnormalities in platelet function can begin early during AKI, before when most clinicians would begin RRT.

Observational studies of AKI using Risk, Injury, Failure, Loss of kidney function and Endstage kidney disease (RIFLE) criteria have provided two important pieces of information: ARF (stage F by RIFLE) is common among critically ill patients (10%–20% of patients in the intensive care unit) and is associated with a 3- to 10-fold increase in the risk of death before discharge. Given the profound increase in the risk of death, many investigators have asked why more patients do not receive RRT, yet many patients with ARF recover renal function without ever receiving RRT. Should these patients receive RRT? Current evidence is insufficient to answer this question, but given the low rates of complications associated with CRRT, and the high risk of death associated with AKI, consideration should be given to starting therapy early (e.g., when stage 3 criteria are present, rather than waiting for complications to occur).

When to Stop RRT

An even more difficult question to answer than when to start is when to stop RRT. Again, the simplest answer is "when renal function has recovered," but two problems exist with this simple answer. First, it is not always easy to determine when renal function has recovered and, second, it is also unclear what amount of recovery should be sought before cessation of therapy. One approach that was used in the largest trial of dialysis intensity published to date used the rule described in Table 6.5. However, attention to fluid and electrolyte status is also required, and most clinicians provide a trial off RRT as opposed to checking creatinine clearance.

Table 6.5 Assessment for recovery of renal function if urine volume is less than 30 mL/h

Creatinine Clearance	Management of RRT
<12 mL/min	Continuation of RRT
12–20 mL/min	Clinician's judgment
>20 mL/min	Discontinuation of RRT

Note: Six hours of timed urine collections need to be obtained for assessment of creatinine clearance. RRT, renal replacement therapy.

Patient Selection for CRRT

Which Patients Should Receive CRRT?

When the decision is made to initiate RRT, the question of which modality (intermittent vs. continuous) arises. The following considerations influence the choice of modality, although, strictly speaking, there are few absolute indications for one modality over the other:

- *Hemodynamic stability*: CRRT is preferred for patients with or at risk for hypotension. In practice, this usually means patients who require vasopressor support either at baseline or as a result of treatment. The ARF Trial Network study demonstrated that hypotension is extremely common with IHD. There is some evidence to suggest that use of CRRT as initial therapy is associated with better recovery of renal function after AKI compared with IHD.
- *Intracranial hypertension*: Intracranial hypertension is an absolute indication for CRRT. IHD induces much greater fluid shifts and is therefore contraindicated in patients with increased intracranial pressure.
- *Severe fluid overload and high obligatory fluid intake*: Even hemodynamically stable patients with severe fluid overload or patients with mild fluid overload but high daily fluid requirements (usually for medications and nutritional support) may be managed more effectively with CRRT. For example, it is unusual to remove more than 3 to 4 L of volume during a 4-hour dialysis session. Yet, it is quite common to remove 200 to 300 mL/h (5–7 L/day) or even more with CRRT.
- *Mechanical ventilation*: For patients who are unable to tolerate weaning trials on nondialysis days, CRRT (or daily dialysis) may be better.
- *High-protein turnover/catabolic patients*: For some critically ill patients, it may be difficult to control solute levels with alternate-day dialysis. Patients with very high predialysis BUN levels may be better treated with CRRT.
- *Hyperkalemia*: When rapid solute clearance is necessary, such as in severe hyperkalemia, intermittent therapy is generally preferred. CRRT is usually quite effective for hyperkalemia, but intermittent therapy is somewhat faster.

Key References

Goldstein S, Bagshaw S, Cecconi M, et al. Pharmacological management of fluid overload. *Br J Anaesth*. 2014;113:756–763.

Hoste EA, Clermont G, Kersten A, et al. RIFLE criteria for acute kidney injury is associated with hospital mortality in critical ill patients: a cohort analysis. *Crit Care*. 2006;10:R73.

KDIGO, AKI Workgroup. Kidney disease: improving global outcomes (KDIGO) clinical practice guideline for acute kidney injury. *Kidney Int*. 2012;2(suppl):1–141.

Rosner MH, Ostermann M, Murugan R, et al. Indications and management of mechanical fluid removal in critical illness. *Br J Anaesth*. 2014;113:764–771.

Palevsky PM, Zhang JH, O'Connor TZ, et al. Intensity of renal support in critically ill patients with acute kidney injury. *N Engl J Med*. 2008.

Tolwani A. Continuous renal-replacement therapy for acute kidney injury. *N Engl J Med*. 2012;367:2505–2514.

Uchino S, Bellomo R, Morimatsu H, et al. Continuous renal replacement therapy: a worldwide practice survey. *Intensive Care Med*. 2007;33(9):1563–1570.

Uchino S, Bellomo R, Morimatsu H, et al. Discontinuation of continuous renal replacement therapy: a prospective multi-center observational study. *Crit Care Med*. 2009;37:2576–2582.

Wald R, Shariff SZ, Adhikari NK, et al. The association between renal replacement therapy modality and long-term outcomes among critically ill adults with acute kidney injury: a retrospective cohort study. *Crit Care Med*. 2014;42:868–877.

Chapter 7

Biomarkers for Initiation of Renal Replacement Therapy

Alexander Zarbock and Lakhmir S. Chawla

Diagnosis of Acute Kidney Injury and Limitations

The diagnosis of acute kidney injury (AKI) is based on changes in serum creatinine levels and/or urine output. However, serum creatinine levels and urine output have a low sensitivity and specificity, respectively. Serum creatinine can be influenced by several factors (e.g., fluid therapy, muscle mass) and it does not reflect kidney function (serum creatinine increases after more than 50% of the glomerular filtration rate is lost) and degree of tubular injury accurately, whereas urine output can be influenced by diuretics and hypovolemia. In addition, both markers cannot predict whether the kidney function improves or deteriorates.

These limitations are thought to account for the poor clinical outcomes associated with AKI. Therefore, the Acute Dialysis Quality Initiative assigned the highest research priority to the discovery and/or standardization of new biomarkers of AKI. In recent years, abundant papers on biomarkers have been published. Most of the studies investigated whether the different biomarkers can detect or predict AKI defined by serum creatinine-based definitions. Several promising studies showed acceptable diagnostic performance for AKI up to 48 hours before a significant change in serum creatinine level. Because available point-of care devices make it possible to measure biomarkers at the bedside within a short time frame (20 minutes), the community has shown great interest in integrating such biomarkers into clinical decision algorithms.

Issues

1. Currently, clinical utility of AKI biomarkers remains largely unevaluated, with the important issue being whether they could improve the management of patients with AKI. Although the early detection of AKI could lead to the implementation of hemodynamic optimization and avoidance of harm, there is still no specific therapeutic option available for treating AKI.
2. In addition, one other important area of potential clinical use is that of guidance in the decision to initiate renal replacement therapy (RRT).

Several studies have investigated whether biomarkers can predict the need for RRT. Next, we review selected publications that have investigated the use of biomarkers for the prediction of subsequent need for RRT.

Biomarker Studies and Need for RRT

Cystatin C

Cystatin C is a 13-kDa nonglycosylated cysteine protease inhibitor produced by all nucleated cells at a constant rate. In healthy subjects, plasma cystatin C is eliminated through glomerular filtration and is metabolized completely by the proximal tubules. Because cystatin C is not secreted in the tubular system, it is normally not found in urine. Therefore, the presence of cystatin C in the urine reflects tubular damage.

Plasma cystatin C is more sensitive in detecting smaller reductions and acute changes in glomerular filtration rate than serum creatinine. However, one has to keep in mind that plasma cystatin C levels can be influenced by immunosuppressive therapy, the presence of inflammation or malignancies, and abnormal thyroid function. Changes in plasma and urine cystatin C can predict AKI. Similar to serum creatinine, knowledge of the baseline is critical to interpretation of these filtration markers.

Several studies investigated whether serum cystatin C can predict the need for RRT in patients with AKI. In all patients, plasma cystatin C was moderately predictive of RRT. In a second analysis excluding patients with an established AKI at admission to the intensive care unit (ICU), plasma cystatin C performed better for RRT prediction.

In 73 patients with established, nonoliguric AKI, of whom 26 required RRT, urine cystatin C and several tubular proteins and enzymes were tested for their prediction of need for RRT. Urine showed a very good diagnostic performance (area under the receiver operating characteristic curve ROC_{AUC}, 0.92; 95% confidence interval [CI], 0.86–0.96). At a cutoff of 1 g/mol creatinine, urine cystatin C had a high sensitivity (92%) and specificity (83%) for predicting RRT. The data on plasma and urine cystatin C in RRT prediction are encouraging, but additional evidence is needed from larger studies before cystatin C can be recommended to use for predicting the need for RRT.

Kidney Injury Molecule 1

Kidney injury molecule 1 (KIM-1) is a type I transmembrane glycoprotein with a cleavable ectodomain (90 kDa). The molecule is localized in the apical membrane of dilated tubules in acute and chronic injury. There are two forms of KIM-1, with only small differences in their C-terminal portion: one is expressed in the kidney, the other in the liver. KIM-1 is believed to play a role in regeneration processes after epithelial injury and in the removal of dead cells in the tubular lumen through phagocytosis.

Liangos and colleagues demonstrated that the ROC_{AUC} for predicting RRT or death for KIM-1 was 0.61 (95% CI, 0.53–0.61), comparable with that of urine output and serum creatinine. In an adjusted analysis, patients in the highest KIM-1 quartile had a higher odds (3.2; 95% CI, 1.4–7.4) for the composite outcome compared with patients with the lowest quartile. However, this was no longer significant in a multivariate analysis. Controversial data exist because KIM-1 was not a significant predictor for RRT in another study.

Neutrophil Gelatinase-Associated Lipocalin

Neutrophil gelatinase-associated lipocalin (NGAL) is a small protein linked to neutrophil gelatinase in specific leukocyte granules. It is also expressed in a variety of epithelial tissues associated with antimicrobial defense. In the normal kidney, only the distal tubules and collecting ducts stain for NGAL expression.

NGAL is upregulated rapidly in the kidney very early after acute injury. The NGAL protein, which can be measured in the blood and in the urine, is one of the earliest and most robustly produced proteins in the kidney after nephrotoxic or ischemic AKI in animal models. Both urine and blood NGAL have been demonstrated to be early predictors of AKI in several clinical scenarios, including trauma, radiocontrast exposure, cardiac surgery, and in critical illness.

Several observational studies have investigated the initiation of RRT using NGAL. Nine of them have been summarized in a recent meta-analysis. In these studies, either urine or plasma/serum NGAL were measured. The incidence of RRT in the included studies was 4.3%. The overall analysis gave an ROC_{AUC} of 0.782 (95% CI, 0.648–0.917) for discriminating patients who would receive RRT associated with AKI. For a cutoff NGAL value of 278 ng/mL, the specificity was 80% and sensitivity was 76%. However, based on the divergent assays and patient populations, it is difficult to translate these findings into a clinically used algorithm.

In a recently published study, the authors found that median urine NGAL levels at the time of enrollment were significantly greater in the patients (17 of 490, 3.5%) in whom RRT was initiated directly (548 ng/mg creatinine [interquartile range, 156–466]) versus the patients (473 of 490, 96.5%) who did not receive acute RRT (61 ng/mg creatinine [interquartile range, 17–232]). No specific cutoff was evaluated, but there was a 2.6-fold increase in the adjusted risk for RRT with increasing urine NGAL levels.

A recently published study investigated urine samples from 1042 adult patients admitted to 15 Finnish ICUs. In this study population, the predictive value of urine NGAL obtained 24 hours after ICU admission for development of AKI was moderate. For RRT, although the predictive value of urine NGAL was good (0.839; 95% CI, 0.797–0.880). The positive likelihood ratio for RRT was 3.81 (95% CI, 3.26–4.47), suggesting that urine NGAL associated well with the initiation of RRT.

Although these data require further confirmation, the existing data on NGAL imply that this biomarker may have an important interaction with conventional criteria to aid in the clinical decision to initiate RRT.

Urine Output after Furosemide Stress Test

Although urine volume is used to diagnose AKI, this marker is unspecific, because it can be influenced by several factors, including hypovolemia and the use of diuretics. A recently published study investigated the ability of a furosemide stress test (FST; one-time dose of 1.0 mg/kg or 1.5 mg/kg depending on prior furosemide exposure) to predict the development of Acute Kidney Injury Network (AKIN) stage III (AKIN-III) in critically ill subjects with early AKI. In this prospective multicenter study, 54 patients were recruited, of whom 25 patients (32.4%) met the primary end point of progression to AKIN-III. Subjects with progressive AKI had significantly lower urine output after an FST in each of the first 6 hours ($P < .001$). The ROC_{AUC} for the total urine output for the first 2 hours after administering an FST to predict progression to AKIN-III was 0.87 ($P = .001$). The ideal cutoff for predicting AKI progression during the first 2 hours after an FST was a urine volume of less than 200 mL (100 mL/h), with a sensitivity of 87.1% and specificity of 84.1%, suggesting that the FST in subjects with early AKI can be used to identify those patients with severe and progressive AKI.

In this same cohort, the investigators assessed the use of an FST with biomarkers and found that they can be used a synergistic fashion. Among the patients in the cohort who had elevated levels of either tissue inhibitor of metalloproteinases (TIMP2)* insulin-like growth factor binding protein 7 (IGFBP7) or NGAL, the ROC_{AUC} value improved from 0.87 to 0.90–0.91. However, future large studies have to confirm these promising findings. If these results can be confirmed in a larger study, this test could be used to answer the unresolved question of when to initiate RRT.

Strategies for Initiation of RRT

Although existing data are encouraging for some biomarkers, there are challenges to create and test biomarker-based strategies for the initiation of RRT. The outcome RRT initiation has the limitation that it is a surrogate outcome, because of the lack of a broad consensus and the wide practice variation in commencing RRT. The decision to initiate RRT is influenced by several factors, including practice of the individual physician, serum creatinine level, urine output, and the overall status of the patient. In addition, such a decision may also be influenced by logistical or organizational issues.

Limitations are as follows:

- Variable timing of sample collection. In some studies the samples were collected at ICU admission, whereas in other studies the samples were acquired at the time of nephrology consultation. In addition, these time points can vary from institution to institution.
- The time between biomarker measurement and initiation of RRT was not stated. Therefore, we cannot judge whether it could help the clinician to initiate RRT "earlier."

- Another issue is that most of the studies do not provide clinically meaningful cutoff values that can be used at the bedside.

The optimal timing of the initiation of has been the focus of studies. The current evidence—derived mainly from observational studies—suggests a trend toward reduced mortality and better renal recovery with earlier initiation of RRT. However, no randomized control trial exists that has demonstrated that the earlier initiation of RRT is associated with a survival or renal recovery benefit. No consensus exists that guides clinicians on this important issue. To test whether the early initiation of RRT is associated with an improved outcome, clinical decision algorithms have to be used that incorporate AKI criteria, patient-specific factors, and biomarkers.

In some studies, early initiation of RRT (Risk, Injury, Failure, Loss of kidney function, and End-stage kidney disease (RIFLE) - Risk or Injury) was associated with a better outcome compared with late initiation of RRT (RIFLE-Failure). However, interpretation of these studies is confounded by the fact that patients who recover renal function or die without receiving RRT were included. One other drawback is that renal support should not be provided for all critically ill patients with mild or moderate AKI, because a considerable proportion of these patients are likely to recover renal function spontaneously and do need RRT. It would be very helpful to identify patients with sustained and severe AKI who will likely need RRT, because this would enable us to start RRT even at milder stages of AKI to provide renal support and to prevent AKI-related complications.

Biomarkers should be incorporated into clinical algorithms that have previously used conventional parameters only, increasing our ability to predict the need for RRT. Future studies have to identify two cutoffs: one that can exclude the need for RRT and another one that identifies a high likelihood of needing RRT. The first cutoff value would identify patients with a mild tubular injury who are likely to recover spontaneously from AKI. The second would aid in the early identification of patients who have persistent and severe renal injury in whom spontaneous renal recovery is unlikely to occur. Depending on the clinical scenario (e.g., cardiac surgery versus ICU patient), these cutoff values may vary. More studies are needed to establish appropriate thresholds and to evaluate this approach in a prospective study.

Summary

Several novel kidney-specific biomarkers have been discovered and described that can be measured in the blood and urine. They can be used for early detection and diagnosis of AKI, when compared with conventional measures of loss of kidney function such as urine output and/or serum creatinine level. However, fewer studies have investigated the potential value of these biomarkers, either alone or in combination with traditional surrogate measures

61

of kidney injury and/or additional clinical factors for early prediction of the need for RRT. Some studies, investigating cystatin C, NGAL, and KIM-1, have suggested these biomarkers can predict which patient will need RRT. If these studies could be confirmed, this would mean these biomarkers have to be incorporated into clinical decision algorithms, because they could enhance our ability to predict the need for RRT. However, given the limitations of the published studies, we cannot adopt their findings into clinical practice today. These limitations include differences in clinical setting (e.g., ICU patients and cardiac surgery patients), type of specimens (urine vs. blood), patient populations, and small sample size.

Because data are currently not sufficient to recommend the routine use of biomarkers for clinical decision making for RRT initiation, additional studies are required. These studies may also help to determine the optimal time point for initiating RRT.

Key References

Bagshaw SM, Cruz, DN, Gibney RT, Ronco C. A proposed algorithm for initiation of renal replacement therapy in adult critically ill patients. *Crit Care.* 2009;13(6):317–324.

Chawla LS, Davison DL, Brasha-Mitchell E, et al. Development and standardization of a furosemide stress test to predict the severity of acute kidney injury. *Crit Care.* 2013;17(5):R207-215.

Gibney N, Hoste E, Burdmann EA, et al. Timing of initiation and discontinuation of renal replacement therapy in AKI: unanswered key questions. *Clin J Am Soc Nephrol.* 2008;3(3):876–880.

Haase M, Bellomo R, Devarajan P, Schlattmann P, Haase-Fielitz A, Ngal Meta-analysis Investigator Group. Accuracy of neutrophil gelatinase-associated lipocalin (NGAL) in diagnosis and prognosis in acute kidney injury: a systematic review and meta-analysis. *Am J Kidney Dis.* 2009;54(6):1012–1024.

Herget-Rosenthal S, Poppen D, Husing J, et al. Prognostic value of tubular proteinuria and enzymuria in nonoliguric acute tubular necrosis. *Clin Chem.* 2004;50(3):552–558.

Liangos O, Perianayagam MC, Vaidya VS, et al. Urinary N-acetyl-beta-(D)-glucosaminidase activity and kidney injury molecule-1 level are associated with adverse outcomes in acute renal failure. *J Am Soc Nephrol.* 2007;18(3):904–912.

Nisula S, Yang R, Kaukonen KM, et al. The urine protein NGAL predicts renal replacement therapy, but not acute kidney injury or 90-day mortality in critically ill adult patients. *Anesth Analg.* 2014;119(1):95–102.

Palevsky PM. Indications and timing of renal replacement therapy in acute kidney injury. *Crit Care Med.* 2008;36(suppl):S224–S228.

Seabra VF, Balk EM, Liangos O, Sosa MA, Cendoroglo M, Jaber BL. Timing of renal replacement therapy initiation in acute renal failure: a meta-analysis. *Am J Kidney Dis.* 2008;52(2):272–284.

Siew ED, Ware LB, Gebretsadik T, et al. Urine neutrophil gelatinase-associated lipocalin moderately predicts acute kidney injury in critically ill adults. *J Am Soc Nephrol.* 2009;20(8):1823–1832.

Chapter 8

Extended Indications

Rinaldo Bellomo and Ian Baldwin

Methods, Techniques, and Approach

Continuous renal replacement therapy (CRRT) can be used to achieve its logical clinical goals in extended indications using different methods. For example, if the issue at stake is that of fluid removal, standard CRRT can be used to lower the urea concentration while aiming for a significant negative fluid balance of −200 to − 400 mL/h. With this approach, large amounts of fluid can be removed from patients with diuretic-resistant fluid overload. If the patient has severe sepsis or septic shock and the goal of therapy is to remove soluble mediators, then either high-volume hemofiltration or high-cutoff hemofiltration can be applied. High-volume hemofiltration requires high blood flows (>300 mL/min) to avoid either excessive predilution (if the replacement fluid is administered before the filter) or excessive hemoconcentration within the filter (if the replacement fluid is administered after the filter). If high-volume hemofiltration is used, attention must be paid to fluid balance and phosphate levels, because relatively minor errors in fluid balance can cause problems when 10 L of fluid are exchanged every hour, and because the rapid removal of phosphate inevitably leads to hypophosphatemia. If high-cutoff hemofiltration (large toxic molecules are the target for removal) is used, special high-cutoff membranes are necessary. High-volume hemofiltration may also be used to remove a water-soluble free toxic drug such as lithium or sodium valproate at higher efficiency than standard CRRT. If this is done, such therapy is best followed by a spell of standard CRRT to avoid the so-called rebound in plasma concentration that follows the cessation of a high-efficiency treatment of blood. In some cases, CRRT can be used to control body temperature in situations such as malignant hyperthermia or severe fever resulting from infection or cerebral injury. In such cases, replacement fluid is not warmed before administration and can even be cooled before administration.

Practical Considerations

The choice to apply CRRT using the techniques just described is based entirely on clinical judgment and a view that the possible benefits of therapy might be greater than its risks. This determination requires that those applying CRRT for extended use should have a very high level of clinical competence in this field so the treatment can be applied with minimal risk. This requirement applies particularly to high-volume hemofiltration, which requires a suitable-quality machine, attention to accurate fluid balance monitoring, frequent monitoring of electrolytes and phosphate, regular phosphate replacement, appropriate adjustment of antibiotic dosage, and attention to body temperature. The risks are much less with severe diuretic refractory fluid overload, especially when secondary to advanced cardiac failure. In such patients, the typical desired fluid removal (10–15 L) can be achieved over 24 to 48 hours by means of a steady negative fluid balance of −300 mL/h. This type of fluid removal is executed easily; it is commonplace during CRRT for acute renal failure, in any case.

For water-soluble drugs with limited or little protein binding and with limited volumes of distribution (<0.5 L/kg), in case of serious life-threatening intoxication, CRRT (perhaps initially at high volume and then, after the levels are within a safe range, at standard volumes) also appears justified, biologically sound, and relatively safe. CRRT has now been used as an adjunctive treatment for

- Sepsis
- Controlling body temperature not responding to conventional approaches
- Decreasing the inflammatory response associated with cardiac arrest
- Achieving or maintaining acid–base homeostasis in patients with severe acidemia
- Removing radiocontrast and attenuating renal injury in patients at risk of radiocontrast nephropathy
- Correcting gross fluid overload of different etiology
- Preventing massive fluid overload in patients receiving large amounts of clotting factors
- Attenuating the inflammatory response associated with prolonged cardiopulmonary bypass
- Correcting sodium disturbances in patients with limited renal function

When all the potential biological, physiological, and clinical effects of CRRT are appreciated, logical use of this therapy outside the field of CRRT is inevitable.

Conclusions for the non-renal or extended uses of CRRT

CRRT has the ability to affect multiple biological and clinical targets. When this ability is appreciated and the technique is mastered, CRRT becomes a tool that can be applied easily to situations outside the simple need for renal replacement therapy. CRRT can lower body temperature, remove fluid, deliver large amounts of buffer, remove water-soluble drugs, affect the inflammatory and counterinflammatory systems, modulate electrolyte concentration, and allow the rapid administration of large amounts of blood products without the associated development of fluid overload. When these properties are appreciated, extended indications for CRRT simply become logical physiological interventions similar to those achieved with mechanical ventilation.

Key References

Atan R, Crosbie D, Bellomo R. Techniques of extracorporeal cytokine removal: a systematic review of the literature. *Blood Purif*. 2012;33:88–100.

Atan R, Virzi GM, Peck L, et al. High cut-off hemofiltration versus standard hemofiltration: a pilot assessment of effects on indices of apoptosis. *Blood Purif*. 2014;37:296–303.

Bellomo R, Baldwin I, Ronco C. High-volume hemofiltration. *Curr Opin Crit Care*. 2000;6:442–445.

Bellomo R, Baldwin I, Ronco C. Rationale for extracorporeal blood purification therapies in sepsis. *Curr Opin Crit Care*. 2000;6:446–450.

Cruz DN, Perazella MA, Bellomo R, et al. Extracorporeal blood purification therapies for prevention of radiocontrast-induced nephropathy. *Am J Kidney Dis*. 2006;48:361–371.

Joannes-Boyau O, Honoré PM, Perez P, et al. High-volume versus standard-volume haemofiltration for septic shock patients with acute kidney injury (IVOIRE study): a multicentre randomized controlled trial. *Intensive Care Med*. 2013;39:1535–1546.

Kellum JA, Bellomo R, Mehta R, Ronco C. Blood purification in non-renal critical illness. *Blood Purif*. 2003;21:6–13.

Chapter 9

Dose Adequacy and Assessment

Zaccaria Ricci and Claudio Ronco

Approximately 5% to 6% of critically ill patients admitted to the intensive care unit develop severe acute kidney injury (AKI) and more than 70% of them receive renal replacement therapy (RRT). The mortality rate for severe AKI has exceeded 50% during the past three decades and it represents an independent risk factor for mortality of critically ill patients. Strategies to improve patient outcome in AKI may include optimization of delivered RRT dose.

Theoretical Aspects of RRT Dose

The conventional view of RRT dose is that it is a measure of the quantity of blood purified by "waste products and toxins" achieved by means of renal replacement. The operative measure of RRT dose is the elimination amount of a representative marker solute. The marker solute, however, does not represent all the solutes that accumulate during AKI, because kinetics and volume of distribution are different for each solute. Thus, its removal during RRT is not necessarily representative of the removal of other solutes. A significant body of data suggests that single-solute marker assessment of dose of dialysis appears to have a clinically meaningful relationship with patient outcome and, therefore, clinical utility.

The amount (dose) of delivered RRT can be described by various terms: efficiency, intensity, frequency, and clinical efficacy. *Efficiency* of RRT is represented by the concept of clearance (K)—in other words, the volume of blood cleared of a given solute over a given time (it is generally expressed as volume over time: milliliters per minute, milliliters per hour, liters per hour, liters per 24 hours, and so on). K does not reflect the overall solute removal rate (mass transfer), but rather removal normalized on serum concentration. Even when K remains stable over time, the removal rate varies if the blood levels of the reference molecule change. During RRT, K depends on solute molecular size, transport modality (convection or diffusion), and circuit operational characteristics (blood flow rate [Q_B], ultrafiltration rate [Q_{UF}], dialysate flow rate [Q_D], filter type and size). Q_B, as a variable in delivering RRT dose, is dependent mainly on vascular access and operational characteristics of machines used in the clinical setting. During convective techniques, Q_{UF} is linked strictly to Q_B by filtration fraction (the fraction of plasma water that is removed from blood by ultrafiltration): it is recommended to keep Q_{UF} to less than $0.2 \times Q_B$. During diffusive techniques, when the Q_D to Q_B ratio exceeds 0.3, it can be estimated that dialysate will not be completely saturated by blood-diffusing solutes. Even if "unperfect" solutes, urea and creatinine blood levels are used to guide treatment dose. During ultrafiltration, the driving pressure jams solutes, such as urea and creatinine, against the membrane and into the pores, depending on the membrane sieving coefficient (SC) for that molecule. SC expresses a dimensionless value and is estimated by the ratio of the concentration of the solutes in the filtrate divided by that in the plasma water, or blood. An SC of 1.0, as is the case for urea and creatinine, demonstrates complete permeability; value of 0 reflects complete rejection. Molecular size more than approximately 12 kDa and diameter of filter pores are the major determinants of SC. The K during convection is measured by the product of Q_{UF} multiplied by SC. Thus, there is a linear relationship between K and Q_{UF}, with SC being the changing variable for different solutes. During diffusion, an analogue linear relationship depends on diffusibility of a solute across the membrane. As a rough estimate, it has been shown that, during continuous, slow efficiency treatments, urea K can be considered a direct expression of Q_{UF} and Q_D. K can be used normally to compare the treatment dose during each dialysis session, but it cannot be used as an absolute dose measure to compare treatments with different time schedules. For example, K is typically greater during intermittent hemodialysis (IHD) than continuous renal replacement therapy (CRRT) and sustained, low-efficiency daily dialysis (SLEDD). This is not surprising because K represents only the instantaneous efficiency of the system. However, mass removal may be greater during SLEDD or CRRT. For this reason, the information about the time span during which K is delivered is fundamental to describing the effective dose of dialysis (intensity).

Intensity of RRT can be defined by the product "Clearance x Time" (Kt; which is measured in milliliters per minute multiplied by 24 hours, liters per hour multiplied by 4 hours, and so on). Kt is more useful than K in comparing various RRTs. However, it does not take into account the size of the pool of solute that needs to be cleared; this requires the dimension of efficacy.

Efficacy of RRT is the effective solute removal outcome resulting from the administration of a given treatment dose to a given patient. It can be described as a fractional clearance of a given solute (Kt/V), where V is the volume of distribution of the marker molecule in the body (about 45 L in a 70 kg adult patient). Kt/V is a dimensionless number and it is an established measure of dialysis dose correlating with medium term (several years) survival in chronic hemodialysis patients (e.g., 3 L/h x 24 h/45 L = 72 L/ 45

L = 1.6) . Urea is typically used as a marker molecule in end-stage kidney disease to guide treatment dose (the volume of distribution of urea [V_{UREA}] is generally considered as equal to patient total body water, which is 60% of patient body weight), and a Kt/V_{UREA} of at least 1.2 is currently recommended for IHD treatments. However, Kt/V_{UREA} application to patients with AKI has not been evaluated rigorously as a result of a major uncertainty about V_{UREA} estimation. Some authors have suggested to express dose as K indexed to patient body weight as an operative measure of daily CRRT. It is now suggested to deliver *no less than* 20 mL/kg/h x 24 hours. If the simplification discussed earlier (K = milliliters per hour = Q_{UF} or Q_D) can be considered acceptable, this CRRT dose might be expressed in a 70-kg patient as about 1500 mL/h or 36 L/day of continuous venovenous hemofiltration (CVVH; Q_{UF} x kilograms x 24 hours) or continuous venovenous hemofiltration dialysis (Q_D x kilograms x 24 hours). Interestingly, applying Kt/V_{UREA} dose assessment methodology in a 70-kg patient, the dosage of 20 mL/kg/h x 24 hours would be equivalent to a Kt/V value of 0.8. Furthermore, it is usually necessary to prescribe a higher dose (e.g., 25–30 mL/kg/h) to ensure that delivery is never less than the 20-mL/kg/h prescription. Nevertheless, so far, several clinical trials have failed to show a one-size-fits-all prescription for RRT, and dialysis dose should always be tailored to each patient. The most important point is never to "underdialize" patients, especially in case of sepsis and hypercatabolism.

Other parameters of dialysis dose include acid–base control, tonicity control, potassium control, magnesium control, calcium and phosphate control, intravascular volume control, extravascular volume control, temperature control, and the avoidance of unwanted side effects associated with the delivery of solute control. These aspects of dose are not currently addressed by any attempt of measure, but should be considered when discussing the prescription of RRT.

Practical Aspects of RRT Dose

Table 9.1 and Table 9.2 provide a potential flow chart that could be followed each time an RRT prescription is indicated.

- Urea volume of distribution V (in liters): patient's body weight (in kilograms) x 0.6
- Estimated fractional clearance (Kt/V_{CALC}): K_{CALC} (in milliliters per minute) x Prescribed treatment time (in minutes)/V (in milliliters)
- A dosage of 25 mL/kg/h corresponds roughly to a (theoretically) optimal Kt/V value of 1.0.
- Filtration fraction calculation (postdilution): Q_R/Q_B x 100; filtration fraction calculation (predilution): $Q_R/Q_B + Q_R$ x 100
- Q_B, blood flow rate; Q_R, replacement solution flow rate; Q_{UF}, ultrafiltration flow rate (Q_{UF}: $Q_R + Q_{UF}^{NET}$); Q_{UF}^{NET}, patient's net fluid loss; Q_D, dialysate solution flow rate

Table 9.1 Example of a possible prescription for a continuous treatment in a 70-kg patient (urea volume, 42 L) during an ideal session of 24 hours (time, 1440 minutes)

	Estimated urea clearance (K_{CALC})	Notes	Value of Q to Obtain 25 mL/kg/h	Value of Q to obtain 1 Kt/V
CVVH postdilution	$K_{CALC} = Q_{UF} = Q_R$	Always keep filtration fraction <20% (Q_B must be five times Q_R)	Q_R: 25 mL/min or 2000 mL/h	Q_R: 29 mL/min or 1750 mL/h
CVVH predilution	$K_{CALC} = \dfrac{Q_{UF}}{1 + \dfrac{Q_R}{Q_B}}$	Filtration fraction computation changes (keep <20%)	For a Q_B of 180 mL/min, Q_R: 30 mL/min or 2500 mL/h	For a Q_B of 200 mL/min, Q_R: 35 mL/min or 2100 mL/h
CVVHD	$K_{CALC} = Q_D$	Keep Q_B at least thrice Q_D	Q_D: 25 mL/min or 2000 mL/h	Q_D: 29 mL/min or 1750 mL/h
CVVHDF postdilution (~50% convective and diffusive K)	$K_{CALC} = Q_R + Q_D$	Consider both notes of CVVH and CVVHD	Q_R: 15 mL/min + Q_D: 10 mL/min	Q_R: 14 mL/min replacement solution + Q_D: 15 mL/min

Net ultrafiltration (patient fluid loss) is considered zero in K_{CALC} for simplicity.

RRT Dose Delivery: Continuous or Intermittent

Originally, K is used to evaluate renal function among disparate individuals whose kidneys, however, are operating 24 hours per day and urea/creatinine blood levels are at a steady state. For this reason, the concept of K is easily applicable to continuous treatments, and its use to describe intermittent therapy efficiency is a sort of "adaptation."

K is typically greater in IHD than in CRRT and SLEDD. However, mass removal may be greater during SLEDD or CRRT because the K is applied for 12/24 hours (Table 9.3).

From a physiological point of view, even if a continuous and an intermittent therapy were prescribed to provide exactly the same marker solute removal, still these two treatments could not be comparable. During continuous treatments, when a relatively low K is applied, a slow but prolonged removal of solutes approaches a pseudo steady-state slope (Figure 9.1). In highly intermittent therapies, the intensive K, limited to 4 to 6 h/day, thrice a week, causes the sawtooth slope in solute removal and the eventual rebound during the

Table 9.2 RRT prescription

Clinical Variables	Operational Variables	Setting
Fluid balance	Net ultrafiltration	Continuous management of a negative balance (100–300 mL/h) is preferred in hemodynamically unstable patients. Complete monitoring (CVC, S-G, arterial line, EKG, pulse oximeter) is recommended.
Adequacy and dose	Clearance/modality	Two thousand to 2500 mL/h K (or 25–30 mL/kg/h) for CRRT, consider first CVVHDF. If IHD is selected, with a minimum dose of 1.2 Kt/V administered at least three times per week. Note that a 4- to 5-hour prescription is usually necessary, and monitoring of delivered Kt/V is recommended.
Acid–base	Solution buffer	Bicarbonate buffered solutions are preferable to lactate buffered solutions in case of lactic acidosis and/or hepatic failure.
Electrolyte	Dialysate/replacement	Consider solutions without K+ in case of severe hyperkalemia. Manage $MgPO_4$ accurately.
Timing	Schedule	Early and intense RRT is suggested.
Protocol	Staff/machine	Well-trained staff should use RRT monitors routinely according to predefined institutional protocols.

CRRT, continuous renal replacement therapy; CVC, central venous catheter; CVVHDF, continuous venovenous hemodiafiltration; EKG: electrocardiogram; IHD, intermittent hemodialysis; Kt/V, XXXX; S-G, Swan Ganz catheter.

time span without treatment. These peaks and valleys of solutes, bicarbonate, electrolytes, plasma osmolarity, and volemia are not physiological and might have a detrimental effect on patient hemodynamic, electrolyte, acid–base and other "osmolar" balances.

Furthermore, in the case of IHD, the intercompartmental transmittance (Kc)—in other words, the variable tendency of different tissues to "release"

Table 9.3

	CRRT	IHD
K (mL/min)	35	200
Urea start (mg/dL)	110	110
Urea end (mg/dL)	90	30
Treatment time (min)	1440	240
Total K (K × time)	50.5	48
Urea removed (g)	25	18

CRRT, continuous renal replacement therapy; IHD, intermittent hemodialysis.

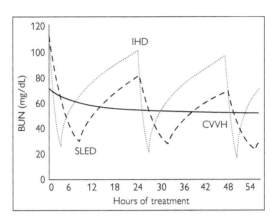

Figure 9.1 Blood urea nitrogen (BUN) patterns over time for intermittent hemodialysis (IHD), continuous venovenous hemofiltration (CVVH), and slow low-efficiency dialysis (SLED).

a solute into the bloodstream—is much more relevant than during long lasting slow efficiency treatments. A system with a low Kc will tend to be less purified during a short dialysis session with respect to another organ with a higher Kc (regardess of treatment intensity). During continuous treatments the Kc will not affect solutes transport into the bloodstream since blood purification will be slow and constant and mainly dependant on tratent intensity.

Different prescriptions may lead to almost equivalent final daily delivery of K. Nonetheless, continuous therapies seem to achieve a final better urea control resulting from the different "physiology" of solute removal (slow, steady, prolonged, and independent from tissue intercompartmental transmittance).

According to recent international surveys on clinical practice patterns, 80% of centers administer CRRT, 17% use intermittent RRT, and a very few apply peritoneal dialysis. Interestingly, in many centers, intermittent techniques are used together with continuous ones, thus evidencing the possibility of multiple prescriptions and practices. Nonetheless, after years of debate, the literature is not able to draw conclusions on how RRT delivery modalities may affect clinical outcomes. Many reports have been published about this issue and they must be analyzed critically.

Many randomized controlled trials compared intermittent and continuous RRT, providing, so far, only conflicting and puzzling results. Based on current scientific evidence, the Surviving Sepsis Campaign guidelines for the management of severe sepsis and septic shock recently concluded that, during AKI, continuous and intermittent dialysis should be considered equivalent evemìn if in hemodynamically unstable patients CRRT might be preferred.

Conclusions

As concluded by the Acute Dialysis Quality Initiative workgroup in 2001, delivered clearance should be monitored during all renal supportive therapies. No recommendations can be made for specific dialysis dosing for patients with specific diseases at this time. A minimum dose of RRT, however, needs to be delivered for AKI:

- The best evidence to date supports the delivery of at least 20 mL/kg/h for CVVH, continuous venovenous hemofiltration dialysis, or continuous venovenous hemodiafiltration. Usually, this requires a target set dose of 25 to 30 mL/kg/h. Currently, there is no evidence of harm in increasing the dose up to 35 mL/kg/h (2–2.5 L/h), which might be beneficial in terms of solute control in selected patients.
- Or 1.2 Kt/V delivered IHD on alternate days. The typically prescribed dose is approximately 1.4 Kt/V for alternate-day dosing.
- For alternate day IHD, isolated ultrafiltration can be used for volume control as needed on nondialysis days.
- It is also recommended that the prescription should exceed that calculated to be "adequate," because of the known gap between prescribed and delivered dose.
- A solute-based approach in the context of dialytic dose may appear restrictive because other dimensions of adequacy of RRT or RRT dose need to be taken in consideration: blood volume control, acid–base control, and tonicity control. However, the solute based-approach of RRT is operatively relatively simple and requires careful attention every time dialysis is prescribed because it allows to monitor the quality and the actual delivery of the treatment.

Key References

Lameire N, van Biesen W, Van Holder R, Colardijn F. The place of intermittent hemodialysis in the treatment of acute renal failure in the ICU patient. *Kidney Int.* 1998;53(suppl):S110–S119.

Ricci Z, Bellomo R, Ronco C. Dose of dialysis in acute renal failure. *Clin J Am Soc Nephrol.* 2006;1:380–388.

Ronco C, Bellomo R, Homel P, et al. Effects of different doses in continuous venovenous haemofiltration on outcomes of acute renal failure: a prospective randomised trial. *Lancet.* 2000;356:26–30.

The VA/NIH Acute Renal Failure Trial Network. Intensity of renal support in critically ill patients with acute kidney injury. *N Engl J Med.* 2008;359:7–20.

Uchino S, Bellomo R, Kellum JA, et al. Patient and kidney survival by dialysis modality in critically ill patients with acute kidney injury. *Int J Artif Organs.* 2007;30:281–292.

Uchino S, Kellum JA, Bellomo R, et al. Acute renal failure in critically ill patients: a multinational, multicenter study. *JAMA.* 2005;294:813–818.

Chapter 10

Acid–Base and Electrolyte Disorders

John A. Kellum

Electrolyte Management

An important principle in the management of electrolytes with continuous renal replacement therapy (CRRT) is that "you get what you replace." With hemofiltration, all electrolytes are removed freely (sieving coefficients near one) and thus, over time and assuming no large intake or other losses, plasma concentrations approach those of the replacement fluid. The rate at which electrolytes change is determined by how different the plasma concentration is relative to that in the replacement fluid and the rate of fluid replacement delivered.

Similar principles exist for continuous hemodialysis, with one exception: phosphate. Although the phosphate molecule is not large, it behaves as if it were a much larger molecule. As a consequence, phosphate is removed much more slowly with hemodialysis (diffusion) compared with hemofiltration (convection). For this reason, patients receiving hemodialysis may still require phosphate binders whereas those receiving hemofiltration frequently require phosphate replacement.

It should be noted that plasma electrolyte concentrations often do not reflect whole-body stores, whereas high or low plasma concentrations still may induce symptoms and deleterious physiological and metabolic effects. In particular, K^+, the primary intracellular cation, exhibits only a loose association between plasma and intracellular concentrations (discussed next). Plasma Mg^{2+} concentrations bear almost no relation to total-body stores, and persistent hypokalemia may be the only clue to total-body Mg^{2+} deficiency.

Electrolytes losses should be considered, as well as electrolyte intake, in prescribing CRRT. An important source of exogenous K^+ is from transfusions of banked blood. Blood transfusions are also an import cause of hypocalcemia because of the citrate anticoagulation used in blood banking. Important sources of electrolyte loss are shown in Table 10.1

Specific fluid-prescribing information for both continuous venovenous hemofiltration and continuous venovenous hemofiltration dialysis is included in Chapter 14.

Table 10.1 Electrolyte losses

Large nasogastric aspirate, vomiting	Na^+, Cl^-
Sweating	Na^+, Cl^-
Polyuria	Na^+, Cl^-, K^+, Mg^{2+}
Diarrhea	Na^+, Cl^-, K^+, Mg^{2+}
Ascitic drainage	Na^+, Cl^-

Dysnatremias

CRRT is rarely required as primary therapy for dysnatremias, but patients with renal failure frequently develop dysnatremia and care must be taken to correct sodium levels according to the rate in which the abnormality has developed and in response to the nature of the symptoms present. In general, dysnatremias that develop slowly should be treated slowly; rapidly occurring dysnatremias demand rapid correction. Severe symptoms also require rapid treatment, although correction is partial, at first, in the case of chronic conditions. Finally, volume status should be considered in the treatment plan.

Hypernatremia

Hypernatremia manifests as thirst, lethargy, coma, seizures, and muscular tremor and rigidity, and an increased risk of intracranial hemorrhage. Thirst usually occurs when the plasma sodium level increases 3 to 4 mmol/L greater than normal. Lack of thirst is associated with central nervous system disease (see Table 10.2).

Rate of correction
- If hyperacute (<12 hour), correction should be rapid.
- Otherwise, aim for gradual correction of plasma sodium levels (over 1–3 days), particularly in chronic cases (>2 days' duration), to avoid cerebral

Table 10.2 Causes of hypernatremia

Type	Etiology	Urine
Low total body Na	Renal losses: diuretic excess, osmotic diuresis (glucose, urea, mannitol)	$[Na^+]$ > 20 mmol/L iso- or hypotonic
	Extrarenal losses: excess sweating	$[Na^+]$ <10 mmol/L hypertonic
Normal total body Na	Renal losses: diabetes insipidus	$[Na^+]$ variable hypo-, iso-, or hypertonic
	Extrarenal losses: respiratory and renal insensible losses	$[Na^+]$ variable hypertonic
Increased Total-body Na	Conn's syndrome, Cushing's syndrome, excess NaCl, hypertonic $NaHCO_3$	$[Na^+]$ >20 mmol/L iso- or hypertonic

edema through sudden lowering of osmolality. A rate of plasma sodium lowering of less than 0.7 mmol/h has been suggested.

Low or normal total body Na (water loss)
- Reduce Na concentration in replacement fluid or dialysate (see Chapter 14 for specific fluids).
- Water replacement by mouth may be given in addition to changes in CRRT fluids.
- Even fluid balance (or even fluid gain with replacement fluid) until total-body water is normalized.
- If central diabetes insipidus (CDI) is present, restrict salt and administer thiazide diuretics. Complete CDI requires desmopressin (10 μg twice daily intranasally or 1–2 μg twice daily intravenously [IV]) whereas partial CDI may require desmopressin but often responds to drugs that increase the rate of ADH secretion or end-organ responsiveness to ADH (e.g., chlor-propamide, hydrochlorothiazide).
- If nephrogenic diabetes insipidus is present, manage with a low-salt diet and thiazides. High-dose desmopressin may be effective. Consider removal of causative agents (e.g., lithium).

Increased total body Na (Na gain)
- Reduce Na concentration in replacement fluid or dialysate (see Chapter 14 for specific fluids).
- Fluid removal is targeted at achieving an even fluid balance or, if hypervol-emia, a net negative fluid balance.

Hyponatremia

Hyponatremia may cause nausea, vomiting, headache, fatigue, weakness, muscular twitching, obtundation, psychosis, seizures, and coma. Symptoms depend on the rate as well as the magnitude of decrease in the plasma [Na^+]. (see Table 10.3)

Rate and degree of correction
- Rate and degree of correction depend on how rapidly the condition has developed and whether the patient is symptomatic. Hyponatremia that has developed over more than 48 hours is considered chronic.
- In *chronic, asymptomatic hyponatremia*, correction should not exceed 4 mmol/24 h and the rate of correction should not exceed 0.3 mmol/L/h.
- In *chronic symptomatic hyponatremia* (e.g., seizures, coma), correction should be 1 to 1.5 mmol/L/h until symptoms resolve, then correct as per asymptomatic cases.
- In *acute hyponatremia* (<48 h), the ideal rate of correction is controversial, although elevations in plasma Na^+ can be faster, but <20 mmol/L/day.
- A plasma Na^+ level of 125 to 130 mmol/L is a reasonable target for initial correction of both acute and chronic states. Attempts to achieve eunatre-mia rapidly should be avoided.

Table 10.3 Causes of hyponatremia

Type	Etiology	Urine [Na⁺]
ECF volume depletion	Renal losses: diuretic excess, osmotic dieresis (glucose, urea, mannitol), renal tubular acidosis, salt-losing nephritis, mineralocorticoid deficiency	>20 mmol/L
	Extrarenal losses vomiting, diarrhea, burns, pancreatitis	<10 mmol/L
Modest ECF volume excess (no edema)	Water intoxication (NB postoperative, TURP syndrome), inappropriate ADH secretion, hypothyroidism, drugs (e.g., carbamazepine, chlorpropamide), glucocorticoid deficiency, pain, stress.	>20 mmol/L
	Acute and chronic renal failure	>20 mmol/L
ECF volume excess (edema)	Nephrotic syndrome, cirrhosis, heart failure	<10 mmol/L

- Neurological complications (e.g., central pontine myelinolysis) are related to the degree of correction and, in chronic hyponatremia, the rate. Premenopausal women are at highest risk for this complication.

Extracellular fluid volume excess
- If symptomatic (e.g., seizures, agitation), 100-mL aliquots of hypertonic (1.8%) saline can be given. Check plasma levels every 2 to 3 hours.
- If symptomatic and edematous, fluid removal on CRRT can be provided in addition to hypertonic saline. Check plasma levels every 2 to 3 hours. With custom replacement fluid or dialysate, the Na concentration can be increased somewhat, but hypertonic dialysis or replacement fluid is not recommended.
- If not symptomatic, restrict water to 1–1.5 L/day. If hyponatremia persists, consider inappropriate ADH [syndrome of inappropriate antidiuretic hormone secretion (SIADH)] secretion.
- If SIADH likely, administer isotonic saline and consider demeclocycline.

Extracellular fluid volume depletion
- If symptomatic (e.g., seizures, agitation), give isotonic (0.9%) saline. Consider hypertonic (1.8%) saline initially, especially if acute.
- If asymptomatic, use isotonic (0.9%) saline.
- Maintain an even fluid balance on CRRT.

General points
- Equations that calculate excess water are unreliable. It is safer to monitor plasma sodium levels closely.
- Hypertonic saline may be dangerous, especially in the elderly and in those with impaired cardiac function.
- Use isotonic solutions for reconstituting drugs, parenteral nutrition, and so forth (i.e., avoid hypotonic fluids).
- Hyponatremia may intensify the cardiac effects of hyperkalemia.

- A true hyponatremia may occur with a normal osmolality in the presence of abnormal solutes (e.g., ethanol, ethylene glycol, glucose).

Causes of Inappropriate ADH Secretion
- Neoplasm, for example, lung, pancreas, lymphoma
- Most pulmonary lesions
- Most central nervous system lesions
- Surgical and emotional stress
- Glucocorticoid and thyroid deficiency
- Idiopathic
- Drugs (e.g., chlorpropamide, carbamazepine, narcotics)

Potassium and Magnesium

Both K^+ and Mg^{2+} are, primarily, intracellular cations. Their total-body concentrations depend on the balance between intake and excretion; their plasma concentrations are determined by total-body stores as well as by their distribution across cell membranes. In the case of K^+, plasma pH and $[Na^+]$ also affect the plasma concentration. Excretion is controlled primarily by the kidneys, although both cations are excreted in the feces as well.

Hyperkalemia
Hyperkalemia may cause dangerous arrhythmias, including cardiac arrest. Arrhythmias are related more closely to the rate of increase in potassium than the absolute level. Clinical features such as paresthesia and areflexic weakness are not clearly related to the degree of hyperkalemia but usually occur after electrocardiographic (EKG) changes (tall T waves, flat P waves, prolonged PR interval, and wide QRS).

Causes
- Reduced renal excretion (e.g., renal failure, adrenal insufficiency, diabetes, potassium-sparing diuretics)
- Intracellular potassium release (e.g., acidosis, rapid transfusion of old blood, cell lysis including rhabdomyolysis, hemolysis, and tumor lysis)
- Potassium poisoning

Management
CRRT is effective in removing K^+, although intermittent hemodialysis can remove K^+ faster. Ancillary therapy may also be required, particularly in emergency situations (see Chapter 6).

Hypokalemia
Typical manifestations of hypokalemia include the following:

- Arrhythmias (SVT, VT, and torsades de pointes)
- EKG changes (ST depression, T-wave flattening, U waves)

- Constipation
- Ileus
- Weakness

Causes
- Inadequate intake
- Gastrointestinal losses (e.g., vomiting, diarrhea, fistula losses)
- Renal losses (e.g., diabetic ketoacidosis, Conn's syndrome, secondary hyper-aldosteronism, Cushing's syndrome, renal tubular acidosis, metabolic alkalosis, hypomagnesemia, drugs including diuretics, steroids, theophyllines)
- Hemofiltration losses
- Potassium transfer into cells (e.g., acute alkalosis, glucose infusion, insulin treatment, familial periodic paralysis)

Management
Potassium replacement should be IV with EKG monitoring when there is a clinically significant arrhythmia (20 mmol over 30 minutes, repeated according to levels). Slower IV replacement (20 mmol over 1 hour) should be used when there are clinical features without arrhythmias. Oral supplementation (to a total intake of 80–120 mmol/day, including nutritional input) can be given when there are no clinical features.

Hypomagnesemia

Magnesium is primarily an intracellular ion involved in the production and use of energy stores, and in the mediation of nerve transmission. Low plasma levels, which do not necessarily reflect either intracellular or whole-body stores, may thus be associated with features related to the following functions:

- Confusion, irritability
- Seizures
- Muscle weakness, lethargy
- Arrhythmias
- Symptoms related to hypocalcemia and hypokalemia that are resistant to calcium and potassium supplementation, respectively

Normal plasma levels range from 1.7 to 2.4 mg/dL; severe symptoms do not usually occur until levels decrease to less than 1.0 mg/dL.

Causes
- Excess loss (e.g., diuretics), other causes of polyuria (including poorly controlled diabetes mellitus), severe diarrhea, prolonged vomiting, large nasogastric aspirates
- Inadequate intake (e.g., starvation), parenteral nutrition, alcoholism, malabsorption syndromes

Management
- For severe, symptomatic hypomagnesemia, 10 mmol magnesium sulfate can be given IV over 3 to 5 min. This administration can be repeated once or twice as necessary.

- In less acute situations or for asymptomatic hypomagnesemia, 1–2 g $MgSO_4$ solution can be given over 1 to 2 hours and repeated as necessary, or according to repeat plasma levels.
- A continuous IV infusion can be given; however, this is usually reserved for therapeutic indications when supranormal plasma levels (4–5 mg/dL) of magnesium are sought (e.g., treatment of supraventricular and ventricular arrhythmias, preeclampsia and eclampsia).
- Oral magnesium sulfate has a laxative effect and may cause severe diarrhea.

Hypermagnesemia

Symptomatic hypermagnesemia rarely occurs even in severe renal failure except as a consequence of a large magnesium load (in which it may occur even with intact renal function). However, patients with renal failure may develop severe hypermagnesemia when exposed to magnesium-containing antacids or laxatives, even in usual therapeutic dosages. Thus, these agents are contraindicated in patients with severe renal failure. Most cases of hypermagnesemia are mild (<3.6 mg/dL, or 1.5 mmol/L) and asymptomatic. However, three types of symptoms may be seen when plasma magnesium concentration exceeds 4.8 mg/dL (2 mmol/L): neuromuscular, cardiovascular, and hypocalcemia (see Table 10.4).

Causes
- IV magnesium infusion (typically as treatment for preeclampsia)
- Oral ingestion (e.g., laxative, Epsom salts)
- Magnesium enemas

Management
Peritoneal dialysis, intermittent renal replacement therapy (RRT), and CRRT have been used effectively to lower the plasma magnesium concentration in patients with severe symptomatic hypermagnesemia, usually in the setting of renal failure complicated by exogenous magnesium loading. Intermittent hemodialysis with its higher flow rates works more rapidly, lowering magnesium levels to the nontoxic range usually within 3 to 4 hours. CRRT is typically slower, and peritoneal dialysis is usually reserved for milder cases in patients

Table 10.4 Relationship of plasma magnesium and clinical symptoms		
Plasma [Mg^{2+}]	**Deep tendon Reflexes**	**Other symptoms/signs**
4.8–7.2 mg/dL (2–3 mmol/L)	Diminished	Nausea, flushing, headache, lethargy, and drowsiness
7.3–12 mg/dL (3–5 mmol/L)	Absent	Somnolence, hypocalcemia, hypotension, bradycardia, and ECG changes
>12 mg/dL (>5 mmol/L)	Absent	Muscle paralysis, respiratory paralysis, complete heart block, and cardiac arrest

receiving chronic peritoneal dialysis. Exchange transfusion has been effective in neonatal hypermagnesemia.

While awaiting dialysis in a patient with severe symptoms, IV calcium can be given as a magnesium antagonist. The usual dose is 100 to 200 mg elemental calcium over 5 to 10 minutes.

Calcium and Phosphate

Ca^{2+} and $PO_3^4$are often considered together in patients with renal failure because a common complication of chronic disease is renal osteodystrophy or bone mineral disease, which leads to hypocalcemia and hyperphosphatemia.

Hypocalcemia

Symptoms of hypocalcemia usually appear when total plasma calcium levels are less than 8 mg/dL and the ionized fraction is below 0.8 mmol/L. Other symptoms are as follows:

- Tetany (including carpopedal spasm)
- Muscular weakness
- Hypotension
- Perioral and peripheral paresthesia
- Chvostek and Trousseau's signs
- Prolonged QT interval
- Seizures

Causes
- Associated with hyperphosphatemia
  - Renal failure
  - Rhabdomyolysis
  - Hypoparathyroidism (including surgery), pseudohypoparathyroidism
- Associated with low/normal phosphate levels:

  - Critical illness including sepsis, burns
  - Hypomagnesemia
  - Pancreatitis
  - Osteomalacia
  - Overhydration
  - Massive blood transfusion (citrate binding)
  - Hyperventilation and the resulting respiratory alkalosis may reduce the ionized plasma calcium fraction and induce clinical features of hypocalcaemia.

Management
- If respiratory alkalosis is present, adjust ventilator settings or, if spontaneously hyperventilating and agitated, calm and/or sedate. Rebreathing into a bag may be beneficial.

- Administer 1 g calcium chloride or 3 g calcium gluconate (270 mg elemental calcium) IV infusion over 30 to 60 minutes.
- If symptomatic, give 5 to 10 mL 10% calcium chloride or 15 to 20 mL 10% calcium gluconate solution over 10 to 15 minutes. Repeat as necessary.
- Correct hypomagnesemia or hypokalemia if present.
- If asymptomatic and in renal failure or hypoparathyroid, consider enteral/parenteral calcium supplementation and vitamin D analogues.
- If hypotensive or cardiac output is decreased after administration of a calcium antagonist, give 5 to 10 mL 10% calcium chloride solution over 2 to 5 minutes.

Hypercalcemia

Among all causes of hypercalcemia, hyperparathyroidism and malignancy are the most common, accounting for greater than 90% of cases.

Symptoms of hypercalcemia usually do not become apparent until the total (ionized + unionized) plasma levels are more than 13 mg/dL (normal range, 8.5–10.5 mg/dL). Symptoms depend on the patient's age, the duration and rate of increase of plasma calcium, and the presence of concurrent medical conditions. Signs and symptoms of hypercalcemia may include the following (see Table 10.5):

- Nausea, vomiting, weight loss, pruritus
- Abdominal pain, constipation, acute pancreatitis
- Muscle weakness, fatigue, lethargy
- Depression, mania, psychosis, drowsiness, coma
- Polyuria, renal calculi, renal failure
- Cardiac arrhythmias

Causes

- Malignancy (e.g., myeloma, bony metastatic disease, hypernephroma)
- Hyperparathyroidism
- Granulomatous disease (e.g., sarcoidosis, tuberculosis)
- Excess intake of calcium, vitamin A or D
- Drugs (e.g., thiazides, lithium)
- Immobilization
- Rarely, thyrotoxicosis, Addison's disease

Table 10.5 **Drug dosage**	
Diuretics	Furosemide 10–40 mg IV every 2–4 hours (may be increased to 80–100 mg IV every 1–2 hours)
Steroids	Hydrocortisone 100 mg qid IV or prednisolone 40–60 mg by mouth for 3–5 days
Pamidronate	15–60 mg Slow IV bolus
Calcitonin	3–4 U/kg IV followed by 4U/kg SC bd

Management
- Identify and treat cause when possible.
- Carefully monitor hemodynamic variables, urine output, and ECG morphology, with frequent estimations of plasma Ca^{2+}, PO_4^{3-}, Mg^{2+}, Na^+, and K^+.
- Intravascular volume repletion inhibits proximal tubular reabsorption of calcium and may lower plasma Ca^{2+} by 1 to 2 mg/dL. It should precede diuretics or any other therapy. Isotonic saline is typically used.
- Calciuresis. After adequate intravascular volume repletion, a forced diuresis with furosemide plus 0.9% saline (6–8 L/day) may be attempted.
- Steroids can be effective for hypercalcemia related to hematological cancers (lymphoma, myeloma), vitamin D overdose, and sarcoidosis.
- Calcitonin has the most rapid onset of action with a nadir often reached within 12 to 24 hours. Its action is limited (usually does not decrease plasma Ca^{2+} by more than 2–3 mg/dL), is usually short-lived, and rebound hypercalcemia may occur.
- Biphosphonates (e.g., pamidronate) and IV phosphate should be given only after other measures have failed, in view of their toxicity and potential complications.
- CRRT or intermittent RRT may be indicated, particularly early on if the patient is in established oligoanuric renal failure and/or is fluid overloaded.
- CRRT or intermittent RRT without calcium in the dialysis or replacement fluid are both effective therapies for hypercalcemia, although they are usually considered treatments of last resort. RRT may be indicated in patients with severe malignancy-associated hypercalcemia and renal failure or heart failure, in whom hydration cannot be administered safely.
- The use of CRRT or intermittent RRT in patients with hypercalcemia but without renal failure may require modification of the composition of dialysis solutions. In one case report, hemodialysis with a dialysis solution containing 4 mg/dL phosphorus resulted in rapid correction of all abnormalities in a patient in whom medical therapy had failed to reverse hypercalcemia, mental status changes, and hypophosphatemia resulting from primary hyperparathyroidism.

Calcium and Phosphate

Hypophosphatemia

Hypophosphatemia is often asymptomatic even when severe (<1 mg/dL). Symptoms may include muscle weakness (including respiratory muscles and can be associated with inability to wean from mechanical ventilation) rhabdomyolysis, paresthesias, hemolysis, platelet dysfunction, and cardiac failure.

Causes
- Critical illness

- Inadequate intake
- Loop diuretic therapy (including low-dose dopamine)
- Parenteral nutrition (levels decrease rapidly during high-dose IV glucose therapy, especially with insulin)
- Alcoholism
- Hyperparathyroidism

Management

Mild hypophosphatemia may be treated with oral phosphate supplements. In severe and symptomatic cases, 20 to 40 mmol of $NaPO_4$ or $KaPO_4$ should be given by IV infusion over 6 hours and repeated according to the plasma phosphate level.

Hyperphosphatemia

Hyperphosphatemia itself does not produce symptoms. The major concern for hyperphosphatemia is the high circulating levels of parathyroid hormone that result and, in turn, its role in the development of renal osteodystrophy and possibly in other uremic complications as well. High levels of plasma Ca^{2+} and PO_4^{3-} together may cause calcinosis (soft-tissue calcifications), especially if the plasma $Ca \times PO_4$ product is chronically less than 70.

Causes

There are three general circumstances, alone or in combination, in which hyperphosphatemia occurs:

1. Massive acute phosphate load (e.g., tumor lysis, rhabdomyolysis)
2. Renal failure
3. Increased phosphate reabsorption (hypoparathyroidism, acromegaly, familial tumoral calcinosis, bisphosphonate therapy, vitamin D toxicity)

Management

The approach to therapy differs in acute and chronic hyperphosphatemia. Acute severe hyperphosphatemia with symptomatic hypocalcemia can be life-threatening. The hyperphosphatemia usually resolves within 6 to 12 hours if renal function is intact. Phosphate excretion can be increased by saline infusion, although this can further reduce the serum calcium concentration by dilution.

CRRT or intermittent RRT are often indicated in patients with symptomatic hypocalcemia, particularly if renal function is impaired. Unlike other electrolytes, phosphate is removed more efficiently with CRRT (in hemofiltration mode) compared with intermittent hemodialysis. This is because PO_4^{3-} acts in solution as a larger molecule and is more difficult to remove with diffusion (dialysis) compared with convection (filtration).

Pseudohyperphosphatemia

Spurious hyperphosphatemia may result from interference with the analytical methods.

Causes
- Hyperglobulinemia, hyperlipidemia, hemolysis, and hyperbilirubinemia
- Liposomal amphotericin B

General Acid–Base Management

Increased intake, altered production, or impaired/excessive excretion of acid or base leads to derangements in blood pH. With time, respiratory and renal adjustments correct the pH toward normality by altering the plasma levels of PCO_2 or strong ions (Na^+, Cl^-).

Increased Intake
- *Acidosis*: Chloride administration (e.g., saline), aspirin overdose
- *Alkalosis*: $NaHCO_3$ administration, antacid abuse, buffered replacement fluid (hemofiltration)

Altered production

- *Increased acid production*: Lactic acidosis, diabetic ketoacidosis

Altered excretion
- Hypercapnic respiratory failure, permissive hypercapnia
- *Alkalosis*: Vomiting, large gastric aspirates, diuretics, hyperaldosteronism, corticosteroids
- *Acidosis*: Diarrhea, small bowel fistula, urethroenterostomy, renal tubular acidosis, renal failure, distal renal tubular acidosis, acetazolamide

General Management Principles
- Correct (when possible) the underlying cause (e.g., hypoperfusion)
- NaCl infusion for vomiting-induced alkalosis; insulin, Na^+, and K^+ in diabetic ketoacidosis
- Correct pH in specific circumstances only (e.g., $NaHCO_3$ in renal failure)
- Avoid large-volume saline-based fluids. Consider lactated Ringer's solution or hetastarch in balanced electrolyte solution (Hextend) for fluid resuscitation.

CRRT Management
- Acid–base abnormalities may be caused by improper use of CRRT (e.g., during citrate anticoagulation) and are amenable to correction with CRRT.
- Correction of plasma pH occurs because of a change in plasma strong ion difference (SID) and, to a small extent, a change in weak acid concentration.

Rules of Thumb for pH Correction with CRRT
- The standard base excess (SBE) quantifies the change in plasma strong ion difference (SID) required to restore pH to 7.4 for a pCO_2 level of 40 mmHg.

For example, an SBE of 10 indicates the SID must be increased by 10 mEq/ L to correct the acid–base abnormality completely.
- To increase SID, increase Na^+ or decrease Cl^- and or lactate.
- To decrease SID, decrease Na^+ or increase Cl^-.
- Do not change Na^+ beyond the normal range (135–145 mEq/L).
- Use "buffer" (bicarbonate or lactate) to increase the difference between Na^+ and Cl^- in the dialysate or replacement fluid.
- Typically, correction of half the abnormality is undertaken, then reassessment is conducted.
- Avoid overcorrection of acid–base abnormalities, particularly in cases of metabolizable acid anions (e.g., lactate, ketones) (see Metabolic Acidosis next).

Metabolic Acidosis

A reduced arterial blood pH with a reduced SID and a base deficit of more than 2m Eq/L. Outcome in critically ill patients has been linked to the severity and duration of metabolic acidosis and hyperlactatemia.

Causes

Lactic acidosis. Can be due to tissue hypoperfusion (e.g., circulatory shock). The anion gap (or strong ion gap) is increased with lactic and other organic acids, and poisons. Anaerobic metabolism contributes in part to this metabolic acidosis; however, other cellular mechanisms are involved and may be more important. Lactic acidosis may be seen with increased muscle activity (e.g., postseizure, respiratory distress). Lung lactate release is seen acute lung injury. High sustained levels suggest tissue necrosis (e.g., bowel, muscle).

- Hyperchloremia (e.g., excessive saline infusion)
- *Ketoacidosis*: High levels of β-hydroxybutyrate and acetoacetate related to uncontrolled diabetes mellitus, starvation, and alcoholism.
- *Renal failure*: Accumulation of organic acids (e.g., sulfuric)
- *Drugs*: In particular, aspirin (salicylic acid) overdose, acetazolamide (carbonic anhydrase inhibition), ammonium chloride. Vasopressor agents may be implicated, possibly by inducing regional ischemia or, in the case of epinephrine, accelerated glycolysis.
- Ingestion of poisons (e.g., paraldehyde, ethylene glycol, methanol)
- Cation loss (e.g., severe diarrhea, small bowel fistulae, large ileostomy losses)

Causes lactic acidosis
- Sepsis
- Acute lung injury
- Diabetes mellitus
- Drugs (e.g., phenformin, metformin, alcohols)

- Circulatory shock (e.g., septic shock, hemorrhage, heart failure)
- Glucose-6-phosphatase deficiency
- Hematological malignancy
- Hepatic failure
- Renal failure
- Short bowel syndrome (D-lactate)
- Thiamine deficiency

Clinical Features
- Dyspnea
- Hemodynamic instability
- A rapidly increasing metabolic acidosis (over minutes to hours) is not the result of renal failure. Other causes, particularly severe tissue hypoperfusion, sepsis, or tissue necrosis should be suspected when there is associated systemic deterioration.

General Management
- The underlying cause should be identified and treated when possible.
- Support ventilation (increase minute volume in controlled mechanical ventilation) to help normalize the arterial pH.
- Reversal of metabolic acidosis is generally an indication of successful therapy. An increasing base deficit suggests the therapeutic maneuvers in operation are either inadequate or wrong.
- The benefits of buffers such as Carbicarb and THAM, or tris-hydroxymethyl-aminomethane, remain unproved.

CRRT Management
- Urgent CRRT/hemodialysis may be necessary, particularly if renal function is also impaired.
- Lactate and ketones are removed easily by CRRT, but they are also metabolized rapidly when the underlying metabolic derangement is reversed. CRRT is rarely the primary therapy for lactic or ketoacidosis.
- Use standard or slightly more alkaline dialysate or replacement fluid. Avoid increasing SID by more than 5 mEq/L because a rapid change in lactate or ketones results in overshoot alkalosis.
- Hyperchloremia does not self-correct in a patient with anuric renal failure. Apart from diet, gastrointestinal losses, and intracellular shifts, the kidney is the primary regulator of plasma electrolytes.
- CRRT is effective in correcting hyperchloremic acidosis.
- Decrease Cl^- in dialysate or replacement fluid by the same interval as the SBE. For example, for an SBE of 10, decrease Cl^- by 10 mEq/L.

Metabolic Alkalosis

An increased arterial blood pH with an increased SID and base excess of more than 2 mEq/L caused either by loss of anions or gain of cations. Because the kidney is usually efficient at regulating the SID, persistence of a metabolic alkalosis usually depends on either renal impairment or a diminished extracellular fluid volume, with severe depletion of K^+ resulting in an inability to reabsorb Cl^- in excess of Na^+.

- The patient is usually asymptomatic, though if spontaneously breathing will hypoventilate.
- A metabolic alkalosis causes a left shift of the oxyhemoglobin curve, reducing oxygen availability to the tissues.
- If severe (pH >7.6), a metabolic alkalosis may result in encephalopathy, seizures, altered coronary arterial blood flow, and decreased cardiac inotropy.

Causes
- Loss of total body fluid, Cl^-, usually as a result of the following:
  - Diuretics
  - Large nasogastric aspirates, vomiting
- Secondary hyperaldosteronism with KCl depletion
- Use of hemofiltration replacement fluid containing excess buffer (e.g., lactate)
- Renal compensation for chronic hypercapnia, which can develop within 1 to 2 weeks. Although more apparent when the patient hyperventilates, or is hyperventilated to normocapnia, an overcompensated metabolic alkalosis can occasionally be seen in the chronic state (i.e., an increased pH in an otherwise stable, long-term hypercapnic patient).
- Excess administration of sodium bicarbonate
- Excess administration of sodium citrate (large blood transfusion)
- Drugs, including laxative abuse, corticosteroids
- Rarely, Cushing's disease, Conn's syndrome, Bartter's syndrome

Management
- Replacement of fluid, Cl^- (i.e., give 0.9% saline), and K^+ losses are often sufficient to restore acid–base balance.
- With distal renal causes related to hyperaldosteronism, addition of spironolactone can be considered.
- Active treatment is rarely necessary. If so, administer 150 mL 1.0 N HCl in 1 L sterile water using a central line. Infuse at a rate not greater than 1 mL/kg/h. Alternatives include oral ammonium chloride or, if the patient has volume overload with intact renal function, acetazolamide 500 mg IV or by mouth every 8 hours.
- Compensation for a long-standing respiratory acidosis, followed by correction of acidosis (e.g., with mechanical ventilation) leads to an uncompensated

metabolic alkalosis. This usually corrects with time, although treatments such as acetazolamide can be considered. Mechanical "hypoventilation" (i.e., maintaining hypercapnia), can also be considered.

CRRT Management

- CRRT is not generally required for management of metabolic alkalosis itself, but in patients receiving CRRT, principles of management of metabolic alkalosis mirror those described earlier for metabolic acidosis.
- If hypernatremia is present, decrease Na^+ in dialysate or replacement fluid.
- Increase Cl^- concentration in dialysate or replacement fluid (increase concentration by the interval of the SBE).
- Metabolic alkalosis can result from regional citrate anticoagulation, particularly if the concentrations of Na^+ and Cl^- are not adjusted. Cl^- concentration should be increased; if using hypertonic sodium citrate, Na^+ concentration in dialysate/replacement fluid should be decreased.
- Avoid citrate and Ca^{++} "dose spirals"; reduce citrate rather than increasing Ca^{++} to avoid citrate overdosing.

Key Reference

Leehey DJ, Ing TS. Correction of hypercalcemia and hypophosphatemia by hemodialysis using a conventional, calcium-containing dialysis solution enriched with phosphorus. *Am J Kidney Dis.* 1997;29(2):288–290.

Part 2

Practice

Chapter 11

Choosing a Renal Replacement Therapy in Acute Kidney Injury

Jorge Cerdá and Claudio Ronco

At the time of choosing a treatment modality for acute kidney injury (AKI), physicians strive to achieve multiple goals (Table 11.1). Most commonly, all goals are hard to achieve simultaneously, and compromises must be made. The choice of renal replacement therapy (RRT) requires a series of decisions (Table 11.2), including RRT modality, membrane characteristics, filter performance, and dialysis delivery (timing, intensity, and adequacy). In this chapter, we "put together" the available evidence and create a realistic framework to assist in the decision-making process. The impact of each of these individual decisions on patient outcomes is discussed in subsequent chapters of this book.

RRT is the last treatment resort when all "conservative" nondialytic therapies have been ineffective. Timing of application, modality of choice, and dose are the main variables to consider. All three variables have recently been objects of research. Although solid evidence has been made available on the adequate dose of RRT, timing and modality remain areas of ongoing controversy.

Discussion has centered not only on the impact of RRT on patient survival, but also, lately, increasing emphasis is being placed on the effects of different RRT modalities on kidney function recovery. Notwithstanding the controversy surrounding large studies, the decision on the application of RRT must remain based on individual patient needs and the resources available at the local level.

Timing

Little evidence informs the decision on optimal timing of initiation of RRT. The decision is quite complex, because it involves patient-related variables (fluid status, diuresis, azotemia, and electrolyte and acid–base status) and process-of-care variables, including available equipment, personnel, and resources.

From an individual patient point of view, the "classic" indications of RRT are obsolete and include severe hyperkalemia, acidosis, or azotemia.

Table 11.1 Characteristics of the "ideal" treatment modality of acute kidney injury in the intensive care unit

Characteristic
Preserves homeostasis
Does not increase comorbidity
Does not worsen patient's underlying condition
Is inexpensive
Is simple to manage
Is not burdensome to intensive care unit staff

Contemporary management strategies in general call for earlier initiation of RRT, before such severe, life-threatening abnormalities have occurred. Transfer of criteria designed for patients with end-stage renal disease (ESRD) to critical patients with AKI has led to a lag in the application of early treatment in clinical practice. Such delay is currently not acceptable; with the technologies currently available, there is no reason why a critically ill patient with AKI should be exposed to avoidable metabolic and fluid complications, which are associated with severe adverse outcomes.

Multiple recent individual studies and meta-analyses suggest that earlier initiation of RRT is beneficial, but difficulties remain on the definition of "early" or "late." Moreover, the subjective nature of the decision and the confounding related to differences between patients who are offered early or late RRT makes interpretation of results difficult.

Design of studies is complex. Current efforts are ongoing to design such a study, which will require a randomized trial that includes a very large number of subjects and clear evaluation of all the variables involved.

Table 11.2 Considerations in renal replacement therapy for acute kidney injury

Consideration	Components	Varieties
Dialysis modality	Intermittent hemodialysis	Daily, every other day, SLED
	Continuous renal replacement therapies	AV, VV
	Peritoneal dialysis	
Dialysis biocompatibility	Membrane characteristics	
Filter performance	Efficiency	
	Flux	
Dialysis delivery	Timing of initiation	Early, late
	Intensity of dialysis	Prescription vs. delivery
	Adequacy of dialysis	Dialysis dose

AV, arteriovenous; SLED, sustained low-efficiency dialysis; VV, venovenous.

New biomarkers have not shown usefulness to determine the right time to initiate RRT. The application of newer AKI staging classifications (such as the RIFLE (Risk, Injury, Failure, Loss and End Stage), AKIN (Acute Kidney Injury Network), and KDIGO (Kidney Disease Improving Global Outcomes) criteria has not been proved to be helpful in determining when to start RRT. Clearly, the best strategy consists of careful individualization of the decision to a specific patient, clinical context, and available resources, and consideration of the demands imposed on the patient and the ability of the patient and his/her kidneys to cope with that demand ("capacity"). All these issues are discussed in detail throughout the book.

Modality

Renal replacement modalities currently in use include intermittent hemodialysis (IHD), continuous renal replacement therapy (CRRT; various forms of application), extended dialysis modalities (extended daily dialysis and prolonged intermittent renal replacement therapy [PIRRT]), and peritoneal dialysis.

The choice of RRT modality is based on patient characteristics and institutional availability. When all options are available, the patient's hemodynamic stability is the main patient characteristic that determines modality choice (Table 11.3). Regardless of the therapeutic goal (fluid removal, control of azotemia, correction of electrolyte or acid–base disorder), there is consensus that

Table 11.3 Indications for specific renal replacement therapies

Therapeutic Goal	Hemodynamics	Preferred Therapy
Fluid removal	Stable	Intermittent isolated ultrafiltration
	Unstable	Slow continuous ultrafiltration
Urea clearance	Stable	Intermittent hemodialysis
	Unstable	CRRT
		Convection: CAVH, CVVH
		Diffusion: CAVHD, CVVHD
		Both: CAVHDF, CVVHDF
Severe hyperkalemia	Stable/unstable	Intermittent hemodialysis
Severe metabolic acidosis	Stable	Intermittent hemodialysis
	Unstable	CRRT
Severe hyperphosphoremia	Stable/Unstable	CRRT
Brain edema	Unstable	CRRT

CAVH, continuous arteriovenous hemofiltration; CAVHD, continuous arteriovenous hemodialysis; CAVHDF, continuous arteriovenous hemodiafiltration; CRRT, continuous renal replacement therapy; CVVH, continuous venovenous hemofiltration; CVVHD, continuous venovenous hemodialysis; CVVHDF, continuous venovenous hemodiafiltration.

hemodynamically unstable patients should be treated with one of the various forms of CRRT. This consensus, not based on randomized control trial results, is reflected in the design of the recent Acute Renal Failure Trial Network (ATN) study (discussed later in this chapter), a randomized study comparing a high versus a lower dose of dialysis, where hemodynamically unstable patients were treated with CRRT, while stable patients were treated with IHD.

The main advantages of IHD include its wide availability and widespread expertise in its application, even in small institutions. Furthermore, IHD is a purely diffusive, fast, generally effective modality that, by nature of high blood and dialysate flows, can rapidly correct abnormalities such as hyperkalemia or water-soluble poisonings. The disadvantages of IHD are also related to its ability to correct abnormalities very fast; often, critically ill patients do not tolerate such fast correction and develop fluid compartment disequilibria with severe consequences, including the onset or worsening of brain edema. When IHD is the only option, modifications in its application—including long, daily treatments; use of dialysis sodium profiling; and reduction in dialysate temperature to less than 37°C—have been shown to be of benefit.

Continuous modalities include methods that use convection, diffusion, or a combination of convection and diffusion to achieve solute clearance (Table 11.4). In simple terms, diffusion occurs when there is flow of solute across a dialysis membrane along a favorable solute gradient concentration. Convection is the movement of solute forced by solvent movement across a hemofilter, driven by a hydraulic pressure gradient ("solvent drag").

An accompanying chapter in this book (Chapter 3) describes recent concepts in RRT nomenclature and kinetics in detail. Briefly, different modalities of

Table 11.4 Advantages and disadvantages of various renal replacement modalities

Modality	Use in Hemodynamically Unstable Patients	Solute Clearance	Volume Control	Anticoagulation
PD	Yes	++	++	No
IHD	Possible	++++	+++	Yes/no
IHF	Possible	+++	+++	Yes/no
Intermittent IHF	Possible	++++	+++	Yes/no
Hybrid techniques	Possible	++++	++++	Yes/no
CVVH	Yes	+++/++++	++++	Yes/no
CVVHD	Yes	+++/++++	++++	Yes/no
CVVHDF	Yes	++++	++++	Yes/no

CVVH, continuous venovenous hemofiltration; CVVHD, continuous venovenous hemodialysis; CVVHDF, continuous venovenous hemodiafiltration; IHD, intermittent hemodialysis; IHF, intermittent hemofiltration; PD, Peritoneal dialysis.

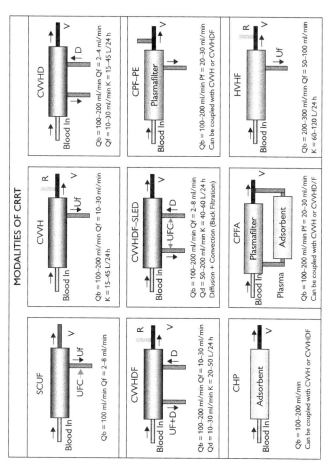

Figure 11.1 Modalities of continuous renal replacement therapy.

Table 11.5 Modalities of continuous renal replacement therapy

Technique	Clearance: Convection*	Mechanism: Diffusion	Vascular Access	Fluid Replacement*
SCUF	+	−	Large vein	0
CAVH	++++	−	Artery and vein	+++
CVVH	++++	−	Large vein	+++
CAVHD	+	++++	Artery and vein	+++
CVVHD	+	++++	Large vein	+/0
CAVHDF	+++	+++	Artery and vein	++
CVVHDF	+++	+++	Large vein	++
CAVHFD	++	++++	Artery and vein	+/0
CVVHFD	++	++++	Large vein	+/0

CAVH, continuous arteriovenous hemofiltration; CAVHD, continuous arteriovenous hemodialysis; CAVHDF, continuous arteriovenous hemodiafiltration; CAVHFD, continuous arteriovenous high-flux hemodialysis; CVVH, continuous venovenous hemofiltration; CVVHD, continuous venovenous hemodialysis; CVVHDF, continuous venovenous hemodiafiltration; CVVHFD, continuous venovenous high-flux hemodialysis; SCUF, slow continuous ultrafiltration.

*0, not required; +, negligible; ++, some; +++, marked; ++++, major.

CRRT (Figure 11.1) are defined by the main mechanism with which clearance is achieved: simple diffusion (continuous hemodialysis, continuous venovenous hemodialysis), convection (continuous hemofiltration, continuous venovenous hemofiltration), or a combination of both (continuous hemodiafiltration, continuous venovenous hemodiafiltration). These different modalities differ in the magnitude of the clearance achieved by convection or diffusion, and the need for fluid replacement (hemofiltration) (Table 11.5).

RRT filters are designated as *dialyzers* when working predominantly in diffusion mode, with a countercurrent flow of blood and dialysate. *Hemofilters* are filters designed to work predominantly in convection mode. In general, these filters have high-flux membranes with high permeability to water and to low- and middle-molecular weight solutes (1000–12,000 Da) and have high "biocompatibility." Newer designs allow the achievement of powerful, simultaneous convection and diffusion (high-flux dialysis, hemodiafiltration).

With current CRRT machines, solute exchange can be obtained by convection, diffusion or both, with easier and more precise control over each component of the therapy. Blood, dialysate, and ultrafiltrate flow rates can be controlled accurately with integrated pumps, and greater dialysate or convective flows—and therefore greater diffusive and convective solute fluxes—can be achieved. In contrast to IHD, during continuous dialysis, diffusion is limited by a low dialysate; the addition of convection improves the clearances of middle-molecular weight solutes (hemodiafiltration). At the slow flow rates usually used with CRRT, there is no interaction between diffusive and convective clearances. Recent studies have shown that the addition of a diffusive component to a convective RRT system (such as in continuous venovenous hemodiafiltration) increases the "dose" of RRT and results in improved survival.

The main advantage of CRRT is that it is applied on a continuous basis, and therefore allows for continuous adjustment of prescription according to the rapidly varying conditions of the critically ill patient. Moreover, although CRRT is a slow technique with lesser blood and dialysate (when applicable) flows, its continuous application effects develop over many hours, and thus—over the long run—CRRT is able to achieve higher solute clearances than IHD.

As opposed to IHD, CRRT (especially when using convective clearance primarily or exclusively) leads to much less or no disequilibria between fluid compartments, and therefore avoids such critical consequences as brain edema—a frequent complication of IHD. It is for this reason that, in the patient with or at risk of brain edema (head trauma, neurosurgery, or patients with liver failure), CRRT is the only modality of choice and IHD should be avoided. Frequent episodes of hypotension during IHD in hemodynamically unstable patients may also contribute to worsened brain edema.

CRRT is associated with better tolerance to fluid removal for a variety of reasons:

1. The rate of fluid removal is much slower in CRRT than in IHD. The main determinant of hemodynamic instability during RRT is the maintenance of intravascular compartment volume. The volume of that compartment is the result of the balance between convective removal of fluid (ultrafiltration) from plasma and the rate of replenishment from the interstitium. Therefore, whenever the ultrafiltration rate exceeds the rate of interstitium-to-plasma flow (refilling), the patient experiences hypovolemia and hemodynamic instability.

2. In IHD, rapid diffusion of urea creates a plasma-to-interstitium and interstitium-to-cell osmotic gradient that drives water to the interstitium and to the intracellular compartment, such that plasma volume decreases and cell edema (including neuronal edema) occurs. With CRRT, the slower rate of urea clearance allows for equalization of urea concentrations between compartments and, therefore, lessened water shifts and cell edema. This is particularly important in patients with intracranial hypertension, such as seen in patients with head trauma and acute liver failure.

3. Commonly, CRRT induces moderate hypothermia. A decrease in core temperature and the resultant peripheral vasoconstriction has been shown to decrease hypotensive episodes and may play a role in hemodynamic stability.

4. With either pre- or postdilution hemofiltration, the magnitude of sodium removal is less than the amount of sodium removed with hemodialysis—a factor that may contribute to better cardiovascular stability in hemofiltration.

5. Although hypovolemia is the first step in dialysis-related hypotension, the ultimate arterial pressure response to hypovolemia is the result of a complex interplay between active and passive mechanisms, including decreased venous vessel capacity to sustain cardiac filling, increased arterial vascular resistance to ensure organ perfusion, and increased myocardial contractility and heart rate to maintain cardiac stroke volume. Any factor interfering with one or more of these compensatory mechanisms may foster cardiovascular instability. In this context, it is possible that convective removal of inflammatory mediators could contribute to hemodynamic stability, especially during the early phases of septic shock.

Recent evidence suggests an advantage in the use of convective techniques (such as continuous venovenous hemofiltration) to remove medium- and large-molecular weight toxins including cytokines and endotoxins. However, more evidence is necessary to demonstrate benefit in a large randomized study; for the moment, no such study has shown a conclusive benefit.

Recent evidence is accumulating on the pharmacokinetics of CRRT, with extensive data informing the use of different medications in CRRT patients. This is especially important because, as a result of the increasing efficiency of newer forms of CRRT, there is a risk that excessive clearance of medications (such as antibiotics) might affect patients adversely.

Much has been made on the problems associated with the prolonged heparin anticoagulation required to maintain a continuous modality. Recent evidence on the clear advantages of citrate anticoagulation on patient survival and acid–base control makes citrate the anticoagulant of choice. Among other reasons for favoring citrate anticoagulation, citrate avoids the complications of continuous heparinization in bleeding-prone critically ill patients.

The cost of CRRT is generally greater than that of IHD or PIRRT. However, cost of RRT must be seen in the context of overall admission costs, especially considering the numbers of days patients spend in the intensive care unit (ICU) and on mechanically assisted ventilation. Seen from this perspective, the overall costs of RRT are quite minor. If the application of CRRT shortens length of stay or time on the ventilator, the impact of CRRT on cost becomes irrelevant.

In an effort to use mixed modalities that resemble IHD, for which there is generally wide proficiency, hybrid modalities have been developed, including sustained low-efficiency dialysis and PIRRT. These hybrid modalities commonly use modified IHD machines with decreased blood and dialysate flow rates to minimize dialysis disequilibrium and hemodynamic instability. Although increasing single-center reports show comparable results with CRRT, these hybrid techniques suffer from a dearth of evidence on what is the adequate dose or what are the clearance characteristics of toxins and medications, and it is therefore difficult, at this time, to reach solid conclusions on patient outcomes in a widely applicable sample.

Despite numerous observational studies, randomized controlled trials, and three systematic reviews and meta-analyses, there is no evidence that any single modality of RRT is associated with improved patient outcome. The inclusive Cochrane meta-analysis found similar hospital and ICU mortality, length of stay, and renal recovery among critically ill patients treated with CRRT or IHD. However, in contrast to how IHD is performed routinely in the "real world", most of these studies applied IHD maximizing hemodynamic tolerance (by increasing duration, daily frequency, positive sodium balance, and thermal adjustments) and the high rate of crossover between treatment modalities makes interpretation difficult. A recent meta-analysis by Schneider shows that, among AKI survivors, initial treatment with IHD may be associated with higher rates of dialysis dependence among survivors, but this finding largely relies on observational trials subject to significant confounding, especially allocation bias by favoring IHD to treat more stable and more chronic kidney disease (CKD) patients.

Two large trials—the ATN and the Randomized Evaluation of Normal versus Augmented Level Renal Replacement Therapy (RENAL)—provided information on the possible impact of choice of RRT on renal recovery. In the ATN trial, in which IHD was delivered 5077 times, 45.2% of survivors required continued dialysis dependence by day 28, whereas in the RENAL trial, in which IHD was used 314 times, dialysis dependence was 13.3% at 28 days. Some of this variation may be dependent on other determinants such as earlier initiation of RRT in the RENAL trial, and differences in patient mix and clinical practice. The recent Kidney Disease Improving Global Outcomes (KDIGO) guidelines recommend the use of CRRT in hemodynamically unstable patients or in patients with brain edema or severe liver failure. In general, around the world, with large geographic differences in practice, CRRT is applied to critically ill patients, and when patients become more stable but still require RRT, those patients are transitioned to IHD. Some evidence suggests that the use of IHD in unstable patients may be associated with worse survival and lesser renal recovery.

In current clinical practice, the choice of RRT modality is based primarily on equipment availability and local expertise on any certain modality. The choice of modality varies widely among countries. In high-income countries, CRRT is the main modality for the treatment of critically ill patients, especially in Europe, Australia, New Zealand, and Canada, but less so in the United States. In low- and middle-income countries, IHD remains the mainstay of treatment, because the use of CRRT is limited by cost and expertise limitations. In low-income countries with limited resources, peritoneal dialysis is used with acceptable results, especially when modified for the critically ill patient.

Dose

The definitions and impact of different doses of RRT on patient outcomes is discussed elsewhere in this book. Results of very well designed randomized controlled trials have demonstrated that a minimal dose of IHD should consist of a weekly Kt/V of 3.9, or a CRRT dose of 20 to 30 mL/kg/h. Despite initial results suggesting benefit of a higher dose, subsequent studies have shown that higher or much higher doses do not lead to better patient outcome. Why this is so is unclear, and may be related to the dialytic and convective losses of valuable nutrients or medications, which leads to lessened survival. It is important to recognize that, realistically, to achieve a minimum of 25 mL/kg/h, it is generally necessary to prescribe a higher dose, usually 30 mL/kg/h, to achieve the dose goal despite multiple discontinuations in CRRT treatment (such as discontinuations due to system clotting, tests, or surgical procedures).

Long-Term Sequelae of AKI

Previously, AKI was widely considered a "one-shot" disease, which led either to death or to function recovery. During the past few years, it has become increasingly evident that, after AKI, de novo development of CKD or worsening of preexisting CKD is quite common. The current increase in incidence of AKI around the world has made AKI a prime contributor to the incidence of new ESRD. The adverse clinical outcomes and the staggering costs of CKD and ESRD have made this interaction an important public health problem, especially in countries with limited health resources. Multiple studies show that AKI should be considered among the classic risk factors for CKD, together with obesity, diabetes, and hypertension. The precise pathophysiological mechanism of progression is unclear.

Several studies have shown an association between the severity of AKI and the risk of subsequent CKD progression. CKD patients who develop AKI have an up to 40 times greater likelihood of progression to ESRD compared with patients with no baseline CKD, whereas patients with CKD but no AKI have an approximately eight times greater risk of ESRD. Although, expectedly, the elderly are at a particular risk for progression to CKD and ESRD, it has been clearly shown that AKI can also be a significant factor of progression to ESRD in children.

Clinical models have been developed in which—by multivariable analysis—variables associated with CKD progression include need for dialysis, baseline estimated glomerular filtration rate (eGFR), serum albumin concentration, and RIFLE stage. Patients who require RRT during AKI have a 500-fold greater risk of CKD compared with those who do not require RRT.

Therefore, RRT management during AKI is likely to have a critical impact on short- and long-term outcomes. As discussed earlier, studies suggest that delayed initiation of RRT may have a negative impact on outcomes, in part by allowing persistence of fluid overload, which has been shown to be a negative factor in kidney recovery. Also, data such as that discussed earlier on RRT modality suggest that CRRT may be associated with better function recovery when compared with IHD, in part because of repeated episodes of intradialytic hypotension in the latter modality. There is no evidence that neither the dose of dialysis nor the use of certain filter membranes has an impact on kidney recovery. Finally, observational data have shown benefit in the use of citrate anticoagulation during CRRT in contrast to heparin or no anticoagulation.

More research is needed in the continuum between AKI and CKD. It is essential to recognize the need to ensure nephrological follow-up of AKI patients after ICU and hospital discharge. Post-AKI interventions will likely have a large impact on the morbidity, mortality, and worsening CKD in this population.

Key References

Askenazi DJ, Selewski DT, Paden ML, et al. Renal replacement therapy in critically ill patients receiving extracorporeal membrane oxygenation. *Clin J Am Soc Nephrol.* 2012;7:1328–1336.

Bellomo R, Kellum JA, Ronco C. Acute kidney injury. *Lancet.* 2012 25;380(9843):756–766.

Cerdá J, Ronco C. Modalities of continuous renal replacement therapy: technical and clinical considerations. *Semin Dial.* 2009;22(2):114–122.

Cerdá J, Tolwani AJ, Warnock DG. Critical care nephrology: management of acid–base disorders with CRRT. *Kidney Int.* 2012;82(1):9–18.

Kellum JA, Lameire N. Diagnosis, evaluation, and management of acute kidney injury: a KDIGO summary (Part 1). Crit Care. 2013;17(1):204

Macedo E, Mehta RL. Timing of dialysis initiation in acute kidney injury and acute-on-chronic renal failure. *Semin Dial.* 2013;26:675–681.

Prowle JR, Kirwan CJ, Bellomo R. Fluid management for the prevention and attenuation of acute kidney injury. *Nat Rev Nephrol.* 2014;10(1):37–47.

Schneider AG, Bellomo R, Bagshaw SM, et al. Choice of renal replacement therapy modality and dialysis dependence after acute kidney injury: a systematic review and meta-analysis. *Intensive Care Med.* 2013;39:987–997.

Tolwani A. Continuous renal-replacement therapy for acute kidney injury. *N Engl J Med.* 2012;367(26):2505–2514.

Chapter 12

Vascular Access for Continuous Renal Replacement Therapy

Alexander Zarbock and Kai Singbartl

Renal replacement therapy (RRT) remains a cornerstone for the management of patients with severe acute kidney injury (AKI). The efficacy of RRT depends on a reliable vascular access.

In critically ill patients, continuous renal replacement therapy (CRRT) is usually performed with a temporary dialysis catheter (TDC), which can be used in any patient, is inserted easily at the bedside, and is used immediately after insertion. Malfunction of the catheter is frequently a result of insufficient blood flow rates, repeated clotting of the extracorporeal circuit, and shortened dialysis time.

Type of Catheter

The demands on TDCs are manifold, including sufficient rigidity to insert the catheter and maintain patency, enough flexibility to prevent kinking, thrombo-resistance, and resistance to bacterial invasion.

Different types of TDCs are available, but CRRT is usually performed with a dual-lumen catheter inserted into a central vein (Figure 12.1). A septum in the catheter separates the two lumina and prevents cross-flow. The two lumina can be arranged side by side or in a concentric manner (coaxial). To minimize the recirculation rate, the tips on the catheter are staged. Frequently, the return tip is longer than the intake tip, with a gap of more than 3 cm separating the two orifices. The choice of the right catheter length, usually 16 cm versus 20 cm, is crucial for both upper body (i.e., internal jugular vein) and lower body (i.e., femoral vein) access sites, because recirculation occurs if the catheter is not long enough.

The two most frequently used blood-compatible materials for dialysis catheters are silicone and polyurethane. The advantage of silicone is that it is soft and flexible, and resistant to most chemicals. However, as a result of its mechanical properties, silicone catheters are more difficult to insert, and compression of the lumen may lead to mechanical failure. On the other hand,

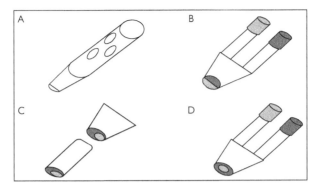

Figure 12.1 Type of catheters used for continuous renal replacement therapy (CRRT). (A) All catheters used for acute CRRT today have tapered tips. Blood is usually removed through the side holes, located at some distance from the tip (~3 cm). (B) The Mahurkar acute dialysis catheter has a so-called *double-D design* that allows blood to be withdrawn through one side of the catheter (intake lumen, dark gray in the figure) and returned through the other side (return lumen, light gray in the figure). (C) The *Circle C catheter* represents a variation of the Mahurkar catheter. Blood is removed through the outer cylindrical lumen and is later returned through the inner cylindrical lumen. Here, the internal surface area is greater than that of the double-D catheter, and therefore resistance to blood flow is greater. (D) The Uldall concentric dual-lumen catheter has an outer surface with side holes in all directions for intake of blood and a concentric inner lumen for blood return through the tip.

the danger of endothelial damage or venous perforation is less. Polyurethane is comparable with silicone with respect to biocompatibility, but it displays a greater tensile strength. A polyurethane catheter can be extruded with a thinner wall, resulting in a larger inner diameter and, subsequently, a greater flow rate, compared with silicon catheters with the same outer diameter. The advantage of polyurethane catheters is that they have thermoplastic properties: rigid during placement, but they soften when soaked at body temperature. The use of polyurethane catheters is often recommended, because it has been shown that this material is associated with reduced bacterial colonization.

Vascular Access Site and Implementation

General Considerations

- The insertion site of the catheter depends on the patient's characteristics (e.g., previous surgery, local infection, coagulopathy, body habitus), the availability of the insertion site, the skill/experience of the operator, and the risks of site-specific complications.
- The Kidney Disease Improving Global Outcomes guidelines recommend using an uncuffed, nontunneled dialysis catheter in patients with AKI.
- As a result of catheter-related bloodstream infection, nontunneled and noncuffed catheters can be used for short-term RRT (<3 weeks), but tunneled

(5–10 cm subcutaneous course) and cuffed catheters should be used if the duration of the RRT is anticipated to be more than 3 weeks.

- TDCs should be inserted using stringent sterile precautions to reduce catheter-related bloodstream infection (CRBSI).
- Ultrasound guidance is recommended to be used for central vein catheterization. This approach can increase the overall success rate and reduce the rate of complications (e.g., hemothorax, pneumothorax, catheter-related infections).
- To check the proper position of the catheter superior vena cava (SVC/right atrium), a chest radiograph promptly after placement and before first use of an internal jugular or subclavian catheter is recommended.
- Preexisting grafts and fistulas in patients with end-stage renal failure should not be used as vascular access sites for TDCs because these catheters can lead to permanent vessel or graft wall damage.

Site of Insertion

Jugular Vein
Insertion in the right internal jugular vein is preferred over the left internal jugular vein because of the increased blood flow and reduced complication rate.

Femoral Vein
The femoral vein is often preferred because of easy and fast accessibility. Transient dialysis catheters in the femoral vein have, for a long time, been thought to be associated with the highest infection rate. A recently conducted multicenter study, however, demonstrated that only in patients with a high body mass index is femoral catheterization associated with an increased infection rate. A recently published meta-analysis analyzing two randomized controlled trials (1006 catheters) and 8 cohort (16,370 catheters) studies also demonstrated that femoral catheterization was not associated with an increased infection rate. Nonetheless, femoral TDCs drastically limit patient mobilization and increase recirculation rates.

Subclavian Vein
The insertion of a central venous catheter in the subclavian vein is accompanied with a low infection rate in critically ill patients. Insertion of a TDC in the subclavian vein is not recommended for patients who may need permanent dialysis access. Subclavian dialysis catheters carry greater rates of central venous stenosis, excluding the ipsilateral arm for future dialysis access. Therefore, the subclavian vein should be reserved for short-term use or when alternative sites are lacking.

Complications

Primary Complications

- Insertion-related complications are arterial puncture, pneumothorax, hemothorax, air embolism, arrhythmias, pericardial tamponade, and retroperitoneal hemorrhage. Most of these complications can be reduced by using ultrasound guidance.

- A reduced blood flow, frequently indicated by increased intake and/or return pressures in the CRRT circuit, are often the result of malpositioning, kinking during insertion, or other mechanical problems. Improper catheter tip placement is a common cause of reduced blood flow and malfunction. Femoral catheters should be inserted in the inferior vena cava, and jugular and subclavian catheters should be placed at the junction of the superior vena cava and the right atrium. Malfunction of catheters in the superior vena cava is decreased further when the tip of the catheters is located in the right atrium, which is safe only with silicone catheters.
- Another problem is the inefficiency of CRRT as a result of recirculation of blood from the return to the intake part of the catheter. This problem arises when the flow generated by the extracorporeal circuit exceeds the flow in the vein. Recirculation rates are normally less than 5% and depend on design, length, and insertion site of the catheter as well as the blood flow in the CRRT circuit.

Secondary Complications

- Infection
  - In intensive care unit patients, risk factors for CRBSI include catheter material, elective versus urgent insertion, the frequency of manipulation, the number of infusion ports, the operator's experience, insertion site, indwelling time, and severity of the underlying illness.
  - Contamination of TDCs can occur as follows: extraluminal contamination (migration of skin flora along the external surface of the catheter into the bloodstream), hematogenous contamination (seeding from another focus of infection), and intraluminal contamination (dominant mechanism in longer dwelling catheters, contamination of the catheter hub through contaminated infusate).
  - The most frequent bacteria are coagulase-negative staphylococci, *Staphylococcus aureus*, enterococci, Gram-negative bacteria, and yeast.
  - TDCs should be used for RRT only.
  - The use of trisodium citrate compared with heparin as a catheter-locking solution reduces catheter-related infections.
  - Using topical antibiotics over the skin insertion site of a nontunneled dialysis catheter in critically ill patients with AKI requiring RRT is not recommended.
  - The use of antibiotic-impregnated catheters prevents CRBSI, but a general recommendation for using these catheters cannot be given because of the emergence of allergic reactions and bacterial resistance.
  - If a clinical suspicion of CRBSI exists, empiric systemic antibiotics appropriate for the suspected organisms should be started after cultures have been grown. After receiving the blood culture results, antibiotic treatment should be tailored to the specific organism.

- A positive result in the culture of the catheter tip necessitates the removal of the catheter and insertion of a new catheter at a new site. However, if an infection at the side of puncture, pocket infection of tunneled catheters, or CRBSI with clinical signs of sepsis exists, the catheter has to be removed immediately.
- Thrombosis

  - Depending on the diagnostic method, the incidence of catheter-related thrombosis may be as high as 33% to 67%.
  - Catheter-related thrombosis may occur as a thrombus adherent to the vessel wall or formation of a fibrin sleeve around the catheter.
  - Catheter-related thrombosis can lead to life-threatening complications, such as right-heart thromboembolism (RHTE) and pulmonary embolism. Nonmobile RHTE originates from the tip of a catheter in the right atrium. Mobile RHTE represents dislodged thrombi from deep venous thromboses in both the upper and lower extremities.
  - During interdialytic periods, the catheter can be filled with an anticoagulant (citrate or heparin) to prevent intraluminal thrombosis.
  - Risk factors for catheter-related thrombosis are listed in Table 12.1.
  - In critically ill patients, the incidence of catheter-related thrombosis is greater for femoral and jugular catheters than subclavian catheters.
- The risk of catheter-related thrombosis and, subsequently, the risk of catheter-related infection can be reduced by administering anticoagulants or by using anticoagulant-bonded catheters.

Table 12.1 Risk factors for temporary dialysis catheter thrombosis

Patient Related	Catheter Related	Site Related
Hypercoagulable states*	Polyurethane/polyvinyl catheters[†]	Femoral or internal jugular site[†]
Thrombophilic states*[†]	Additional central venous catheters simultaneously[†]	Subclavian site*
Age >64 years[†]	Traumatic insertion[†]	
Underlying malignancy*[†]	Distal placement*	
Dehydration[†]		
Impaired tissue perfusion[†]		
Absent prophylaxis/ treatment[†]		

*Associated with right-heart thromboembolism.

[†]Associated with central venous thrombosis.

Source: Modified after Burns KEA, McLaren A. A critical review of thromboembolic complications associated with central venous catheters. *Can J Anesth.* 2008;55:532–541.

Key References

Cimochowski GE, Worley E, Rutherford WE, Sartain J, Blondin J, Harter H. Superiority of the internal jugular over the subclavian access for temporary dialysis. *Nephron.* 1990;54:154–161.

Karakitsos D, Labropoulos N, De Groot E, et al. Real-time ultrasound-guided catheterisation of the internal jugular vein: a prospective comparison with the landmark technique in critical care patients. *Crit Care.* 2006;10:R162.

KDIGO AKI Work Group. KDIGO clinical practice guideline for acute kidney injury. *Kidney Int.* 2012;(suppl 2):1–138.

Marik PE, Flemmer M, Harrison W. The risk of catheter-related bloodstream infection with femoral venous catheters as compared to subclavian and internal jugular venous catheters: a systematic review of the literature and meta-analysis. *Crit Care Med.* 2012;40(8):2479–2485.

NKF-K/DOQI. Clinical practice guidelines for vascular access: update 2000. *Am J Kidney Dis.* 2001;37(suppl 1):S137–S181.

O'Grady NP, et al. Guidelines for the prevention of intravascular catheter-related infections. *Infect Control Hosp Epidemiol.* 2002;23:759–769.

Schillinger F, Schillinger D, Montagnac R, Milcent T. Post catheterisation vein stenosis in haemodialysis: comparative angiographic study of 50 subclavian and 50 internal jugular accesses. *Nephrol Dial Transplant.* 1991;6:722–724.

Vascular Access Work Group. Clinical practice guidelines for vascular access. *Am J Kidney Dis.* 2006;48(suppl 1):S176–S247.

Wentling AG. Hemodialysis catheters: materials, design and manufacturing. *Contrib Nephrol.* 2004;142:112–127.

Chapter 13

The Circuit and the Prescription

Rinaldo Bellomo and Ian Baldwin

Methods and approach

There is no evidence to suggest that choosing continuous renal replacement therapy (CRRT) based on hemofiltration over hemodiafiltration or over hemodialysis leads to clinically important differences in outcomes. There is a clear difference, however, in terms of the nature of solute removal, with convection (filtration) leading to essentially equal small solute removal but much greater middle-molecular weight solute removal. It is unclear, however, whether this effect matters pathophysiologically or clinically. Because of such uncertainty, physicians and nurses choose a particular approach in a given unit (typically based on local tradition, comfort, ease of operation, and so on) and apply it consistently to all patients. Epidemiological data suggest that continuous venovenous hemodiafiltration (CVVHDF) with replacement fluid delivered in pre and or postdilution mode may be the most common approach to CRRT worldwide, followed by continuous venovenous hemofiltration with variable predilution. More important than the choice of modality may be the actual dose delivered (see Chapter 8). The dose depends not only on modality, but also on the size of the patient and the rate of effluent generation.

Practical Considerations

For many machines, CRRT circuits are typically already set up for a particular modality. Thus, when an intensive care unit clinician group has chosen a machine and the modality it wishes to apply to patients, then the appropriate circuit is used during the machine setup. When this is not the case, appropriately designed tubing is typically provided that can be connected to achieve the necessary circuit design. The circuit is then primed with a crystalloid solution (in neonates or small children, the circuit prime might require blood or a blood–albumin mix) and connected to the vascular access catheter. The outflow lumen of the access catheter ("arterial" lumen) is typically labeled in red. The inflow lumen of the catheter is typically labeled in blue ("venous" lumen). If CVVHDF is being implemented, the bag(s) containing suitable replacement

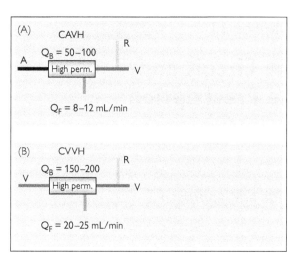

Figure 13.1 (A, B) Diagram of a continuous arteriovenous hemofiltration (CAVH) (A) and a continuous venovenous hemodialysis (CVVH) (B) circuit. A, artery; high perm., high-permeability filter; Q_B, blood flow; Q_F, ultrafiltrate flow; R, replacement fluid; V, vein.

or dialysis fluid is connected to peristaltic roller pumps, which can deliver some of the fluid in the predilution position as replacement fluid (typically 50%) and can also deliver some of the fluid (the other 50%) in a countercurrent direction to blood on the nonblood side of the membrane. However, some machines and circuit design prohibit predilutional CVVHDF because of the reduced diffusive clearance as this dilutes the blood entering the membrane. Finally, the effluent port of the filter is connected with tubing to another peristaltic pump that sets the effluent flow rate. This is typically greater than the sum of the replacement fluid flow rate and the dialysate flow rate to ensure some fluid removal, which compensates for additional fluids (nutrition, drugs, blood products) the patient may be receiving for the care and treatment in the ICU (Figures 13.1, 13.2, 13.3).

When all tubing is connected, the blood pump can be started. This is best done at low flows (especially for patients who require vasopressor support) because, at the start, blood is removed and crystalloid is administered to replace it. This results in the equivalent of acute venesection or "bleed" equal to the volume of the circuit (close to 150 mL in adults) before "pure" blood can both leave and enter the patient at an equivalent rate. Accordingly, the blood pump is best set at 20 to 30 mL/min until the full circuit is primed with blood. When this has happened, gentle increases of 50 mL/min are appropriate until the target flow is achieved. After the blood path has been "set," then therapy (dialysate flow, replacement fluid flow, and effluent generation) can begin. A possible prescription for such therapy is summarized in Table 13.1.

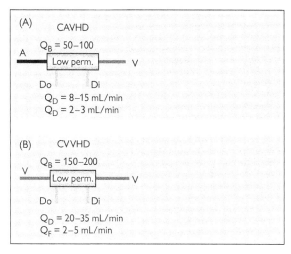

Figure 13.2 (A, B) Diagram of a continuous arteriovenous hemodialysis (CAVHD) (A) and a continuous venovenous hemodialysis (CVVHD) (B) circuit. A, artery; Di, dialysate inflow port; Do, dialysate outflow port; High perm., high permeability filter; Q_B, blood flow; Q_D, dialysate flow rate; Q_F, ultrafiltrate flow; R, replacement fluid; V, vein.

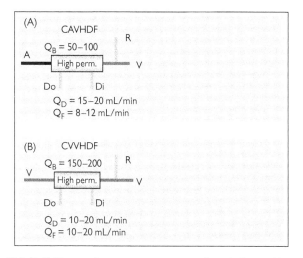

Figure 13.3 (A, B) Diagram of a continuous arteriovenous hemodiafiltration (CAVHDF))(A) and a continuous venovenous hemodiafiltration (CVVHDF) (B) circuit. A, artery; Di, dialysate inflow port; Do, dialysate outflow port; High perm., high permeability filter; Q_B, blood flow; Q_D, dialysate flow rate; Q_F, ultrafiltrate flow; R, replacement fluid; V, vein.

Table 13.1 Prescription for continuous venovenous hemodiafiltration (100 mL/h negative fluid balance)

Patient	Medical Record No.	Technique	Replace-ment Fluid Rate	Dialysate Flow Rate	Effluent Flow Rate	Comments
H. Jones	678945	Continuous venovenous hemodia-filtration	900 mL/h	1000 mL/h	2000 mL/h (25 mL/ kg/h) 100 mL/h fluid loss	Start pump at 30 mL/min and increase to 200 mL/ min over >5 min.

Expected Outcomes, Potential Problems, Cautions, and Benefits

If the principles of circuit design and function are understood, if the consequences of different techniques are appreciated, and if the impact of choosing predilution versus postdilution or both are clear, then the physician can prescribe a logical approach to starting and delivering CRRT and the nurse can conduct CRRT with insight and expertise. This combination of knowledge and expertise inevitably leads to safe and effective delivery of CRRT, which has the following benefits: reliable and safe control of uremia, adequate filter life and costing, complete control of fluid balance, and minimal technical problems. The clinical outcome is a patient in whom CRRT goes on silently and problem-free in the background in a way that is similar to successful mechanical ventilation.

Problems may appear to arise in specific circumstances. However, understanding of the basics will help deal with problems successfully and rapidly. For example, filter life may be short. E.g. less than four hrs use before clotting. If so, assessment of the circumstances surrounding filter loss should allow prevention of similar events.

• Was the patient agitated and flexing the hip in the presence of a femoral vascular access catheter? If so, acute blockage to flow may have been responsible.
• Was the outflow pressure very negative (−120 mmHg) from the very start of therapy? If so, vascular access dysfunction/clotting should be suspected.
• Was the transmembrane pressure low (90–100 mmHg) at the start but increased progressively over 4 to 5 hours of therapy? If so, rapidly progressive filter clotting should be suspected and the circuit anticoagulation approach reviewed.
• Was the dosage correct? Did the assay reflect adequate dosing? Did the postfilter pressure increase while the transmembrane pressure did not change much? If so, one should suspect postfilter obstruction in the air chamber, where clot can frequently form.

All these diagnostic thoughts are logical and derive from understanding the circuit and its components.

Key summary for understanding the circuit in relation to prescribing a therapy with variants of CRRT

The extracorporeal circuit used for CRRT has key components that, if understood clearly, allow physicians to prescribe physiologically logical therapy, and nurses to conduct smooth, safe, and problem-free treatment.

Appreciation of the consequence of choosing a particular technique is important. Understanding of the impact of predilution and postdilution on solute clearance and the effect of blood dilution is similarly important. A clear and logical understanding of pressure measurements along the CRRT circuit is extremely useful in troubleshooting and in making the correct etiological diagnosis when the circuit fails. To conduct CRRT without such knowledge and understanding likely makes the treatment less safe for the patient, less effective in terms of uremic control, and a burden for nurses to develop expertise.

Key References

Baldwin I, Bellomo R, Koch B. A technique for the monitoring of blood flow during continuous hemofiltration. *Intensive Care Med.* 2002;28:1361–1364.

Baldwin I, Tan HK, Bridge N, Bellomo R. Possible strategies to prolong filter life during hemofiltration: three controlled studies. *Renal Fail.* 2002;24:839–848.

Fealy N, Baldwin I, Bellomo R. The effect of circuit "down-time" on uraemic control during continuous veno-venous haemofiltration. *Crit Care and Resusc.* 2002;4:170–172.

Tan HK, Bridge N, Baldwin I, Bellomo R. Ex-vivo evaluation of vascular catheters for continuous hemofiltration. *Renal Fail.* 2002;24:755–762.

Tan CS, Tan HK, Choong HL Real-time circuit pressures correlate poorly with circuit longevity in anticoagulant-free, predilution continuous veno-venous hemofiltration. *Blood Purif.* 2011;32:15–20.

Uchino S, Fealy N, Baldwin I, Morimatsu H, Bellomo R. Continuous is not continuous: the incidence and impact of circuit "down-time" on uremic control during continuous veno-venous hemofiltration. *Intensive Care Med.* 2003;29:1672–1678.

Chapter 14

The Membrane

Size and Material

Zhongping Huang, Jeffrey J. Letteri, Claudio Ronco, and William R. Clark

Hollow Fiber Membranes Used for CRRT: Biomaterial Considerations

As opposed to chronic hemodialysis, for which cellulosic membranes continue to be used, membrane continuous renal replacement therapy (CRRT) filters are almost exclusively synthetic. Synthetic membranes were developed essentially in response to concerns related to the narrow scope of solute removal and the pronounced complement activation associated with unmodified cellulosic filters. The AN69 membrane, a copolymer of acrylonitrile and an anionic sulfonate group, was first used in flat sheet form in a closed-loop dialysate system during the early 1970s for chronic hemodialysis. Since that time, a number of other synthetic membranes have been developed, including polysulfone, polyamide, polymethylmethacrylate, polyethersulfone, and polyarylethersulfone/polyamide. As is the case in chronic hemodialysis, all these membranes have either been used or are currently being used in a CRRT application.

Synthetic membranes are manufactured polymers that are classified as thermoplastics. In fact, for most of the synthetic membranes, the renal market represents only a small fraction of their entire industrial use. With wall thickness values of at least 20 μm, synthetic membranes tend to be thicker than their cellulosic counterparts and, from a structural perspective, they may be symmetric (e.g., AN69, polymethylmethacrylate) or asymmetric (e.g., polysulfone, polyamide, polyethersulfone, polyamide/polyarylethersulfone). In the latter category, a very thin "skin" (approximately 1 μm) contacting the blood compartment lumen acts primarily as the membrane's separative element with regard to solute removal. The structure of the remaining wall thickness ("stroma"), which determines the thermal, chemical, and mechanical properties, varies considerably among the different synthetic membranes.

Although biocompatibility encompasses several different considerations, complement activation has traditionally been the primary parameter used for comparisons of different membranes. As suggested, synthetic membranes as a class result in less complement activation than cellulosic membranes. Because complement activation is roughly proportional to the balance between hydrophilicity (which promotes complement activation) and hydrophobicity (which attenuates complement activation), the relatively hydrophobic nature of synthetic membranes is a benefit in this regard.

Another distinguishing feature of synthetic membranes is their propensity to adsorb plasma proteins. As discussed in more detail later in this chapter, exposure of an extracorporeal membrane to blood results in the instantaneous adsorption of a protein layer ("secondary membrane") that modifies the permeability properties of the native membrane. The composition of this secondary membrane is dominated by relatively high-molecular weight proteins that have the highest plasma concentrations, such as albumin, immunoglobulins, and fibrinogen. However, certain membranes also have the specific capability to remove low-molecular weight (LMW) proteins—such as anaphylatoxins and other inflammatory mediators including cytokines—in significant amounts by adsorption.

With respect to adsorptive removal of LMW proteins, the AN69 membrane (a component of extracorporeal circuits used with the Prisma and Prismaflex CRRT systems) has been studied most widely. Previous investigations have had several findings. First, although the overall secondary membrane formation occurs at the "nominal" (nonpore) membrane surface, the bulk of LMW protein adsorption occurs within the membrane's internal pore structure. Second, the removal of some LMW proteins by AN69 filters occurs exclusively by adsorption, although the molecular weights of such compounds theoretically would allow transmembrane removal. Third, adsorptive removal of LMW proteins by AN69 filters is a saturable phenomenon, usually within the first 60 to 90 minutes of use of a particular filter. Subsequent to saturation, the removal of a specific compound may effectively cease or continue to occur by a "breakthrough" transmembrane mechanism.

Relationship between Ultrafiltration Rate and Transmembrane Pressure in CRRT

Extracorporeal membranes used for dialysis are classified according to their ultrafiltration coefficient as high flux or low flux. However, considerable confusion regarding the exact meaning of flux currently exists. The hydraulic flux of a membrane is the volumetric rate (normalized to surface area) at which ultrafiltration occurs. The clinical parameter used to characterize the water permeability of a specific filter is the ultrafiltration coefficient (K_{UF}, which is measured in milliliters per hour per millimeters mercury). The K_{UF} of a filter is usually derived from in vitro experiments in which bovine blood is ultrafiltered at varying transmembrane pressure (TMP). The membrane characteristic with the largest impact on water permeability is pore size, such that ultrafiltration flux is roughly proportional to the fourth power of the mean membrane pore radius. As such, small changes in pore size have a very large effect on water permeability.

The method by which K_{UF} is determined can be derived from Figure 14.1, in which the relationship between Q_{UF} and TMP is shown for a particular CRRT filter operated under different conditions. The line in the left part of the figure represents the relationship between these two parameters for a "virgin" filter (i.e., no prior exposure to blood or other protein-containing solution) when the test fluid is also an aqueous solution. The slope of the line represents the K_{UF} of the filter for these operating conditions. This strictly linear relationship can be contrasted with the nature of the curve in the right part of the figure. The latter defines a filter's Q_{UF} versus TMP relationship under the condition of ultrafiltration of blood. As the figure indicates, two distinct regions of this curve can be identified: a region controlled by the permeability of the filter membrane itself ("membrane control") and a region controlled by the effects of the secondary membrane on filter performance. (Note that the term *concentration polarization*, which is used in the figure, is essentially synonymous with *secondary membrane* for the purpose of this discussion.)

The membrane control region of the curve occurs at relatively low TMP values and is linear. Similar to the situation of aqueous ultrafiltration with a virgin filter, the slope of the line in this region is the K_{UF} of the filter. The lower slope (i.e., lower K_{UF}) of the right-hand curve is a direct result of the permeability

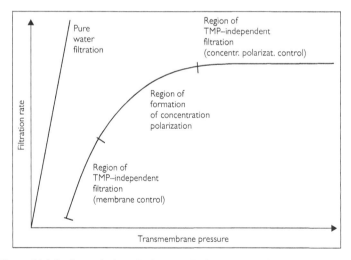

Figure 14.1 Fundamental relationship between ultrafiltration rate and transmembrane pressure (TMP) during ultrafiltration under different operating conditions.

Source: Goehl H, Konstantin P. Membranes and filter for hemofiltration. In: Henderson LW, Quellhorst EA, Baldamus CA, Lysaght MJ, eds. *Hemofiltration*. 1st ed. Berlin: Springer-Verlag; 1986: 73. Reprinted with permission.

reduction resulting from the secondary membrane. As TMP increases, the curve eventually plateaus in the region of secondary membrane control at a certain maximum Q_{UF}, where further increases in TMP result in no additional increase in Q_{UF}. In terms of clinical operation of a filter, the plateau portion of the curve is to be avoided because of the high likelihood of impaired performance or premature clotting of the filter.

As mentioned previously, filter K_{UF} is a value that is specific to a certain set of flow operating conditions, including blood flow rate (Q_B), which influences the nature of the right-hand curve in two ways. First, as Q_B increases, the slope of the curve in the linear (low-TMP) region increases. Effectively, this means to achieve a certain Q_{UF}, a lower TMP is required. The second way in which Q_B influences the nature of these curves is its effect on the maximum achievable (plateau) Q_{UF} such that an increase in Q_B results in a corresponding increase in plateau Q_{UF}.

The explanation for these phenomena is related to the effect of higher Q_B in preserving filter membrane function. Specifically, as Q_B increases, a greater shear force is applied to the proteins comprising the secondary membrane. In this way, the secondary membrane is disrupted and its negative impact on membrane permeability is blunted.

Effect of Secondary Membrane Formation on Solute Permeability in CRRT

The adsorbed protein layer comprising the secondary membrane also reduces the effective solute permeability of a CRRT membrane by "plugging" or blocking a certain percentage of membrane pores. The effect of this process on solute permeability for a polyamide membrane is shown in Figure 14.2. In this

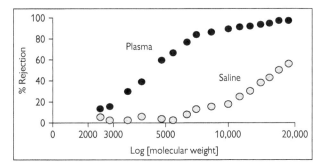

Figure 14.2 Effect of secondary membrane formation on the sieving properties of a polyamide filter membrane.

Source: Feldhoff P, Turnham T, Klein E. Effect of plasma proteins on the sieving spectra of hemofilters. *Artif Organs.* 1984;8:488 Reprinted with permission.

figure, percent rejection, which is essentially equal to one less the sieving coefficient, is plotted against solute molecular weight. Results for both a protein-containing fluid (plasma) and a protein-free fluid (saline) are shown. For a test solute with a molecular weight of 5000 Da, the percent rejection in saline is 0% (i.e., the sieving coefficient is 1.0). On the other hand, for that same solute, the percent rejection in plasma is approximately 60% (sieving coefficient of 0.4).

The adsorptive tendency of a particular membrane varies according to the operating conditions used. Postdilution tends to promote protein adsorption because protein concentrations are higher within the membrane fibers (resulting from hemoconcentration). On the other hand, as mentioned previously, higher Q_B values work to attenuate this process because the shear effect created by the blood disrupts the binding of proteins to the membrane surface.

Membrane Surface Area Effects in CRRT

Early in the era of venovenous CRRT, typical blood and effluent flow rates were less than 150 mL/min and 1.5 L/h, respectively. In this context, filters with surface areas in the range of 0.3 to 0.5 m^2 could generally provide desired solute clearances at acceptable filter operating conditions. However, as blood and fluid flow rates have increased substantially over the years, with the goal of increasing delivered CRRT dose, filter membrane surface area requirements have also increased. For adequate filter operation, the surface area required to provide an effluent-based CRRT dosage target of 35 mL/kg/h is approximately 1.0 m^2 and may be as high as 1.5 m^2 in some larger patients treated with effluent rates greater than 4 L/h.

Continuous Hemofiltration

As discussed earlier, the choice of operating conditions for a hemofiltration procedure should avoid operation of the filter in the secondary membrane-limited region of the Q_{UF}-versus-TMP curve. The clinical corollary of this is the need to select a filter with a surface area that is adequate to support the operating conditions chosen. In Figure 14.3, the relationship between Q_{UF} and Q_B for three theoretical filters of 0.3 m^2, 1.0 m^2, and 1.5 m^2 at constant TMP is shown. In general, these curves have similar contours, with an initial linear region at relatively low Q_B followed eventually by a plateau or quasi-plateau region at relatively high Q_B.

Both the slope of the linear phase and the maximum (plateau) Q_{UF} for each curve are directly proportional to membrane surface area at a given TMP. At a low Q_B (e.g., 75 mL/min), all three filters can generate a relatively low Q_{UF} (e.g., 1.5 L/h) at the same TMP, as denoted by point A on the graph. However, when the clinical goal is a higher Q_{UF} (e.g., 4.0 L/h), a 0.3-m^2 filter is not adequate because the plateau Q_{UF} for this filter falls below the desired value. On the other hand, the higher Q_{UF} is in the operating range of both of the larger filters for the TMP that has been chosen. However, the 1.5-m^2 filter

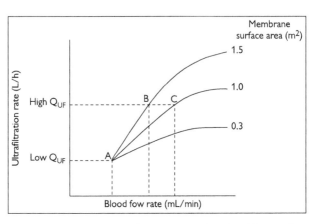

Figure 14.3 Relationship between ultrafiltration rate (Q_{UF}) and blood flow rate for theoretical filters of different surface area. (See the text for an explanation of the operating conditions corresponding to points A, B, and C.)

can achieve this Q_{UF} at a lower Q_B (point B) compared with the 1.0-m^2 filter (point C). An analogous point is that, for a given Q_B, filter membrane surface area is inversely proportional to the TMP required to achieve a certain Q_{UF}.

The general relationship between Q_{UF} and Q_B during hemofiltration described in Figure 14.3 is explained by the phenomenon of filtration pressure equilibrium. In this situation, hydrostatic pressure driving filtration out of the blood compartment is balanced by the oncotic pressure opposing filtration in this direction. When a scenario of filtration pressure equilibrium situation occurs for a filter, surface area is relatively unimportant because the additional surface area is not used for filtration. The corollary is that the benefit of higher surface area on filtration rate can be achieved only if higher Q_B values are used.

Continuous Hemodialysis

Relative to conventional hemodialysis, in which solute clearance is dictated primarily by Q_B and membrane surface area, effluent dialysate flow rate (Q_D) is the primary determinant of solute clearance in continuous venovenous hemodialysis. At least with respect to small-solute clearance, saturation of the effluent indicates optimal use of the prescribed dialysate volume. If such saturation is not achieved, the most likely explanation is a filter of inadequate membrane surface area. When continuous venovenous hemodialysis is performed with a relatively small surface area hemodialyzer (<0.5 m^2), saturation of the dialysate is only achieved at relatively low Q_D values. For a 0.4-m^2 AN69 hemodialyzer, Bonnardeaux and colleagues showed saturation of the dialysate for urea and creatinine is preserved only up to a Q_D of approximately 16.7 mL/min (1 L/h). For Q_D values in the 2- to 3-L/h range (33.3–50 mL/min), although an increase in Q_D resulted in an increase in clearance, a divergence between the

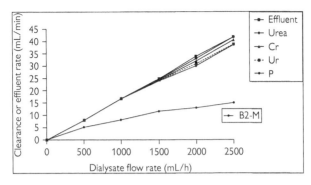

Figure 14.4 Relationship between solute clearance and dialysate flow rate for a 0.9-m² filter in continuous venovenous hemodialysis. B2-M, beta2-microglobulin; Cr, creatinine; P, phosphate; Ur, urate.

Source: Brunet S, Leblanc M, Geadah D, Parent D, Courteau S, Cardinal J. Diffusive and convective solute clearances during continuous renal replacement therapy at various dialysate and ultrafiltration flow rates. *Am J Kidney Dis*. 1999;34:486–492. Reprinted with permission, p. 7

urea/creatinine clearance and the effluent flow rates was observed, indicating nonsaturation of the dialysate. Of course, the greater the degree of nonsaturation, the more inefficient the procedure.

A more contemporary study involving a larger surface area AN69 hemodialyzer (0.9 m²) demonstrates clearly the important effect of surface area on preserving dialysate saturation (Figure 14.4). For this larger hemodialyzer, preservation of effluent dialysate saturation was achieved essentially over the entire Q_D range, the only exception being beta2-microglobulin. The high molecular weight of this compound (approximately 200 times that of urea) severely limits its diffusive capabilities and, therefore, its ability to saturate the dialysate.

Special Membranes and Filters

Most considerations presented thus far deal with standard treatments and materials. Recently, innovations in the field of biomaterials have led to potential use of new filters and devices. Among them, membranes with a functionalized surface to make them more biocompatible, less thrombogenic, and biologically reactive have been developed. This is the case for high-cutoff membranes created to increase clearance of large solutes and chemical mediators, vitamin E-bonded membranes used potentially to reduce oxidant stress, and surface-treated membranes to reduce the amount of anticoagulation and prolong the filter life span, with or without pore opening, for extended clearance capabilities.

Summary Conclusions

In this chapter, an overview of membranes used for CRRT was provided. The major characteristics of hollow fiber membranes influencing both biocompatibility and solute and water removal were described. It is hoped this information provides clinicians with a rational approach to the prescription of CRRT from the perspective of the extracorporeal membrane.

Key References

Bonnardeaux A, Pichette V, Ouimet D, Geadeh D, Habel F, Cardinal J. Solute clearances with high dialysate flow rates and glucose absorption from the dialysate in continuous arteriovenous hemodialysis. *Am J Kidney Dis*. 1992;19:31–38.

Brunet S, Leblanc M, Geadah D, Parent D, Courteau S, Cardinal J. Diffusive and convective solute clearances during continuous renal replacement therapy at various dialysate and ultrafiltration flow rates. *Am J Kidney Dis*. 1999;34:486–492.

Clark WR, Hamburger RJ, Lysaght MJ. Effect of membrane composition and structure on performance and biocompatibility in hemodialysis. *Kidney Int*. 1999;56:2005–2015.

Clark WR, Macias WL, Molitoris A, Wang NHL. Plasma protein adsorption to highly permeable hemodialysis membranes. *Kidney Int*. 1995;48:481–488.

Feldhoff P, Turnham T, Klein E. Effect of plasma proteins on the sieving spectra of hemofilters. *Artif Organs*. 1984;8:186–192.

Goehl H, Konstantin P. Membranes and filter for hemofiltration. In: Henderson LW, Quellhorst EA, Baldamus CA, Lysaght MJ, eds. *Hemofiltration*. 1st ed. Berlin: Springer-Verlag; 1986:: pp. 73–74.

Honore PM, Jacobs R, Joannes-Boyau O, et al. Newly designed CRRT membranes for sepsis and SIRS: a pragmatic approach for bedside intensivists summarizing the more recent advances: a systematic structured review. *ASAIO J*. 2013;59(2):99–106.

Panagiotou A, Nalesso F, Zanella M, et al. Antioxidant dialytic approach with vitamin E-coated membranes. *Contrib Nephrol*. 2011;171:101–106.

Villa G, Zaragoza JJ, Sharma A, Neri M, De Gaudio AR, Ronco C. Cytokine removal with high cut-off membrane: review of literature. *Blood Purif*. 2014;38(3–4):167–173.

Chapter 15

Fluids for Continuous Renal Replacement Therapy

Paul M. Palevsky and John A. Kellum

General Considerations

Considerable variability exists in the prescription of dialysate and replacement fluids for continuous renal replacement therapy (CRRT). In general, the electrolyte composition of these fluids should resemble the physiological composition of plasma water, albeit sometimes with lower potassium and slightly higher buffer content to permit correction of hyperkalemia and metabolic acidosis. Intravenous replacement fluids must be sterile and pyrogen-free. Although dialysate does not need to meet the same standards for sterility, commercially manufactured dialysate for CRRT must be sterile bacteriologically to have a viable shelf-life. Thus, in general, commercially produced fluids are manufactured to the same standards for microbiological purity and may be used safely and interchangeably, whether labeled for use as dialysate or replacement fluid. Before the ready availability of commercially prepared fluids for CRRT, dialysate and replacement fluids were often prepared locally by the hospital pharmacy or at the point of care by the nursing staff. However, this practice has been associated with catastrophic compounding errors and should be discouraged. If fluids are prepared locally, their electrolyte composition should be assayed before use to verify no errors in compounding have been made.

Recommendations for the composition of fluids for CRRT have been published by the Acute Dialysis Quality Initiative and in the Kidney Disease Improving Global Outcomes *Clinical Practice Guidelines for Acute Kidney Injury* and are summarized in the next section.

Electrolyte Composition

Available evidence shows the following:

- Sodium is generally kept at an isonatric (physiological) concentration except when special prescriptions are used in combination with some citrate anticoagulation protocols or during management of hypo- or hypernatremia.

- Potassium, calcium, and magnesium needs are variable in different clinical situations.
- *Phosphate*: Hypophosphatemia resulting from increased clearance and intracellular shifts from refeeding are common in CRRT and may place patients at risk of complications, including muscle weakness and rhabdomyolysis.
- *Glucose*: Maintenance of normoglycemia has been shown to be associated with lesser mortality in critically ill patients. Supraphysiological glucose concentrations in fluids for CRRT should be avoided.
- Trace elements, including water-soluble metals, micronutrients, amino acids, and folate, are lost during CRRT.

Recommendations are as follows:

- *Sodium*: Physiological concentrations should be used except when using citrate anticoagulation. In the latter circumstances, adjustments may be necessary, given the variable contents of sodium in different citrate solutions. Adjustment of the sodium concentration of fluids may also be necessary in patients with hypo- or hypernatremia to achieve an appropriate controlled correction of the serum sodium concentration.
- *Potassium*: Potassium concentrations need to be adjusted over time to maintain serum potassium levels within the normal range. Subphysiological potassium concentrations may be required for the management of hyperkalemia. In patients with gastrointestinal potassium losses, potassium supplementation may be required.
- *Calcium*: Calcium should be present in replacement fluids and dialysate, and should be at approximately physiological concentrations (corresponding to the normal blood ionized calcium). Augmented levels may be necessary in the setting of severe hypocalcemia, and reduced levels may be required in the setting of hypercalcemia. When citrate is used as an anticoagulant, dialysate and replacement fluid containing very low or no calcium are often used; in this setting, an infusion of intravenous calcium is used to replace calcium lost in the effluent to maintain a normal serum ionized calcium concentration.
- *Magnesium*: Dialysate and replacement fluids should contain sufficient magnesium to maintain serum levels in the physiological range.
- *Phosphate*: To avoid hypophosphatemia, phosphate should be provided either as a supplement in the CRRT fluids (replacement fluid and/or dialysate) or provided as intravenous replacement after hyperphosphatemia, if present, has resolved.
- *Chloride*: The chloride concentration of the fluids for CRRT is generally determined by the difference between the concentrations of the cations (sodium, potassium, calcium, magnesium) and the other anions (phosphate and buffers) to maintain electrical neutrality of the solutions.
- *Glucose*: To avoid hyperglycemia, glucose can either be absent or present at physiological concentrations in replacement fluids and dialysate. The use of fluids with supraphysiological glucose concentrations should be avoided.

- *Trace elements*: Losses of trace elements (water-soluble metals, micronutrients, amino acids, and folate) must be appropriately replaced.

Buffer Composition

Lactate Versus Bicarbonate

Both lactate and bicarbonate ions have been used in replacement fluid and dialysate for CRRT. Historically, lactate was been used preferentially as a buffer because of the instability of bicarbonate-based solutions when stored in gas-permeable plastic bags over prolonged periods of time. This problem has recently been overcome, allowing commercial availability of bicarbonate-based fluids. Controlled (although not all randomized) trials have suggested that lactate- and bicarbonate-buffered solutions have a similar efficacy for correction of metabolic acidosis during CRRT. However, recent studies showed better control of metabolic acidosis with bicarbonate compared with lactate.

Blood levels of lactate may be higher when lactate is used in high concentrations (e.g., >10 mmol/L) in replacement fluid (particularly at high volume) and may confuse the clinical interpretation of blood lactate measurements. It is not clear whether this hyperlactatemia is associated with increased morbidity or mortality risk. Depending on tissue redox status and substrate availability, lactate is either metabolized back to pyruvate and into the citric acid cycle or into glucose by gluconeogenesis. Potential concerns with excessive lactate accumulation are hemodynamic compromise, increased urea generation, and cerebral dysfunction. Hyperlactatemia may develop in situations of impaired lactate clearance, including liver failure and tissue hypoperfusion. This hyperlactatemia can be expected to be more pronounced if lactate-buffered solutions are used during high-volume hemofiltration. Accumulation of the D-isomer of lactate may also be a concern because the D-isomer constitutes 50% of the total lactate contents of racemic mixtures. Because humans are not able to metabolize D-lactate, it may accumulate, leading to severely elevated levels, which are associated with neurological impairment.

Acetate

In the intermittent hemodialysis literature, acetate has been shown to be associated with impaired myocardial contractility and decreased cardiac function. This anion has been used rarely as a buffer in CRRT.

Citrate

Used primarily for its anticoagulant properties, citrate serves as an effective buffer. Scant evidence is available on the use of citrate exclusively as a buffer in CRRT. More important, citrate metabolism is often impaired in liver failure or muscle hypoperfusion, with both situations posing risk of hypercitratemia when citrate is used. Hypercitratemia carries the risk of decreased ionized extracellular calcium concentration. More important, blood products contain citrate as an anticoagulant; massive blood or plasma product transfusions are associated with high citrate loads, which accumulate when citrate is used simultaneously as an anticoagulant and a buffer. Low concentrations of citrate are present in some commercial dialysate solutions for intermittent hemodialysis. Complications of citrate toxicity have not been associated with these agents.

Recommendations for use include the following:

- Bicarbonate is an effective buffer and is currently the preferred organic buffer in commercially manufactured solutions.
- Lactate-buffered solutions are safe and efficacious in the majority of patients, but these solutions may be hazardous whenever lactate clearance is impaired, such as in patients with liver failure or severe tissue hypoperfusion. D-Lactate should be removed from lactate-containing solutions, which should consist almost exclusively of L-lactate.
- There are insufficient data to evaluate the use of acetate-buffered solutions in CRRT. However, limited evidence does not support its use compared with lactate or bicarbonate, given the risks of cardiac depression.
- The metabolism of sodium citrate used for regional anticoagulation during CRRT generates 3 mol bicarbonate/1 mol citrate and functions as an efficacious organic buffer. Use of citrate in the setting of decreased citrate clearance or when patients receive large doses of citrate during massive transfusions should be done with individualized adjustment of citrate dose and with close monitoring of plasma ionized calcium levels.

Fluid Prescriptions during Permissive Hypercapnia

In patients with acute respiratory distress syndrome/acute lung injury on lung-protecting ventilator strategies, the resulting respiratory acidosis can be compensated partially or completely by elevation of plasma bicarbonate with CRRT. The decision about the level to which the pH should be corrected is controversial, but most recommend avoiding severe acidosis (pH <7.20).

Example Fluid Orders for CRRT

Keeping in mind that, after a period of equilibration, plasma composition approaches the electrolyte composition of the dialysate or replacement fluid used (with the exception of bicarbonate), the standard composition of CRRT fluids is physiological. Table 15.1 shows various solutions that can be used as either dialysate or as replacement fluids for hemofiltration. Example A might be appropriate for a patient with relatively stable electrolyte and

Table 15.1 Example fluids for CRRT

Fluid	Example A	Example B	Example C
Sodium	140 mEq/L	140 mEq/L	140 mEq/L
Potassium	4 mEq/L	0 mEq/L	4 mEq/L
Chloride	113 mEq/L	109 mEq/L	120.5 mEq/L
Calcium	2.5 mEq/L	2.5 mEq/L	0 mEq/L
Magnesium	1.5 mEq/L	1.5 mEq/L	1.5 mEq/L
Bicarbonate	32 mEq/L	32 mEq/L	22 mEq/L
Lactate	3 mEq/L	3 mEq/L	3 mEq/L
Glucose	100 mg/dL	100 mg/dL	100 mg/dL

acid–base status. Example B might be more appropriate for a hyperkalemic patient. Caution is noted when potassium-free solutions are used to ensure that iatrogenic hypokalemia does not ensue; supplemental potassium can be added to this solution that contains no potassium to achieve a desired final potassium concentration. Example C contains no calcium and has a reduced buffer concentration, and could be used in conjunction with citrate anticoagulation.

Fluid Compounding

Occasionally, severe abnormalities in electrolyte and acid–base balance call for more drastic changes in fluid composition than can be achieved using commercially available solutions. For example, a patient with severe acidosis and hyperkalemia might require a potassium-free solution with a higher concentration of bicarbonate. Although use of a "custom" fluid can be considered, serious errors have been reported when local pharmacies compound fluids without monitoring of composition. Thus, testing should be done on compounded fluids to ensure that errors in composition are not present. Given the varied compositions of commercially available fluids currently available, compounding of "custom" fluids is generally not required. Supplementation of standard fluids with additional electrolytes can also provide a degree of customization. For example, using strict protocols, sodium or potassium phosphate may be added to prevent phosphate depletion and obviate the need for intravenous phosphate replacement. Similarly, the sodium concentration can be adjusted by adding hypertonic sodium chloride; however, strict protocols should be followed and the final sodium concentration monitored. In patients with severe acidemia, short-term bicarbonate supplementation can be provided by using a solution of 150 mEq sodium bicarbonate in 1 L sterile water as additional replacement fluid. In each of these situations, close monitoring of the patient's electrolyte and acid–base status is mandatory.

Summary

The electrolyte composition of fluids for CRRT should generally approximate that of normal plasma, but should be adjusted as necessary to accommodate each patient's needs. Both lactate and bicarbonate are able to correct metabolic acidosis in most CRRT patients; however, correction of acidosis may not be as efficient with lactate as with equimolar bicarbonate. Worsening hyperlactatemia has been noted when lactate was used in patients with lactic acidosis or liver failure. The clinical relevance of this finding is unknown. Thus, bicarbonate is the preferred buffer, especially in patients with lactic acidosis and/or liver failure, and when high-volume hemofiltration is used. However, lactate is an effective buffer in most CRRT patients.

Citrate used as an anticoagulant has also been used effectively as a buffer in CRRT. When citrate is used as an anticoagulant, the concentrations of other buffers need to be adjusted or eliminated, depending on the specific regimen, to minimize the risk of iatrogenic metabolic alkalosis. Monitoring of plasma pH and ionized calcium is required.

Key References

Culley CM, Bernardo JF, Gross PR, et al. Implementing a standardized safety procedure for continuous renal replacement therapy solutions. *Am J Health Syst Pharm.* 2006;63(8):756–763.

Davenport A. Replacement and dialysate fluids for patients with acute renal failure treated by continuous veno-venous haemofiltration and/or haemodiafiltration. *Contrib Nephrol.* 2004;144:317–328.

Kellum JA, Cerda J, Kaplan LJ, Nadim MK, Palevsky PM. Fluids for prevention and management of acute kidney injury. *Int J Artif Organs.* 2008;31(2):96–110.

Kellum JA, Mehta R, Angus DC, Palevsky P, Ronco C, ADQI Workgroup. The First International Consensus Conference on Continuous Renal Replacement Therapy. *Kidney Int.* 2002;62(5):1855–1863.

Kidney Disease: Improving Global Outcomes (KDIGO) Acute Kidney Injury Work Group. KDIGO clinical practice guideline for acute kidney injury. *Kidney Int.* 2012;2(suppl):1–138.

Kierdorf H, Leue C, Heintz B, Riehl J, Melzer H, Sieberth HG. Continuous venovenous hemofiltration in acute renal failure: is a bicarbonate—or lactate-buffered substitution better? *Contrib Nephrol.* 1995;116:38–47.

Leblanc M, Moreno L, Robinson OP, Tapolyai M, Paganini EP. Bicarbonate dialysate for continuous renal replacement therapy in intensive care unit patients with acute renal failure. *Am J Kidney Dis.* 1995;26(6):910–917.

Chapter 16

Alarms and Troubleshooting

Zaccaria Ricci, Ian Baldwin, and Claudio Ronco

Training

Intensive care unit (ICU) physicians and nurses involved in the prescription and delivery of continuous renal replacement therapy (CRRT) operate safely and best with protocols and defined procedures. The following is a list of key aims for training and education.

- An educational program providing theoretical content is necessary.
- A training program for practical skills specific to using CRRT is also necessary, with a connection to the theory.
- All training should be sequenced to provide a logical flow that embraces the cycle of use from preparation of a CRRT machine, patient connection and management during use, and then cessation of treatment (i.e., disconnection).
- Programs need to be continuous and repeated as a result of the ongoing technological developments and high staff turnover.
- A simple simulator can be achieved by placing a double-lumen access catheter into a 5-L saline bag, simulating the patient for machine connection.
- It is desirable to have the majority of staff working at a "competent" level with small groups at the "novice" and "expert" levels. Novice practitioners can also be assisted and supervised by expert colleagues.

Vascular Access

Venovenous CRRT relies on the use of a temporary double-lumen catheter, typically inserted into one of the central veins (femoral, subclavian, or jugular). Ideal catheter type, size, and site of insertion are determined by local hospital policies; however, success can be achieved with many variations and no controlled data are available to reflect "best" practice. Catheters should be easy to insert and remove or be able to be guidewire exchanged, allow a wide range of blood flows, minimize recirculation phenomena, and reduce decubitus and infection episodes. Key considerations for access catheter use are as follows:

- *Catheter type and size*: Double-lumen catheters, as a general rule, can be classified into short (about 15 cm) and long (more than 20 cm), and small (<11 Fr) and big (>13 Fr). The catheter lumen design profile varies, but all designs can obstruct by contact with vessel walls and or kinking resulting from body positional changes during nursing.
- *Catheter site*: Jugular venous catheterization access does not appear to reduce the risk of infection compared with femoral access, except among adults with a high body mass index, and may have a higher risk of hematoma. The site of catheter placement should depend on clinician skill, the presence of other central venous catheters, and the risk of bleeding. Insertion of the catheter to the right atrium promotes reliable use and higher blood flow rate.
- *Catheter troubleshooting*: A malfunctioning catheter is suspected when CRRT monitor pressure alarms occur as low "arterial" or high "venous." The catheter could be guidewire exchanged; however, this is not always successful to resolve the problem and a new site insertion is necessary. Swapping over the connections to the CRRT circuit may also resolve the catheter malfunction but creates a recirculation of blood. This may not be of clinical consequence when solute levels are in control and can allow treatment to continue when fluid balance is the key goal, and a new access catheter insertion is not done easily.
- The catheter should be inserted with the use of ultrasonographic guidance possibly choosing the vessel whose diameter is 1/3 of catheter size.

Circuit Pressures

Modern-technology CRRT machines allow continuous pressure measurement and display for both operator (human) and "smart software" (machine) interpretation. This requires measurement from several different points in the circuit:

- Machine access (negative) pressure and return (positive) pressure depend mostly on the performance of vascular access relative to programmed blood flow rate and patient position.
- *Inlet of the filter*: This pressure indicates the resistance of blood that is pumped into the filter. The gradient of filter inlet and catheter return is defined as "drop pressure" (DP) and is generally calculated automatically by all modern monitors. DP indicates the capacity of blood to flow through the membrane.
- *Effluent/ultrafiltrate port pressure*: This value can be positive when the filter is new or spontaneous ultrafiltration (UF) occurs. When the filter pores are being reduced in size and number as a result of clotting, UF occurs only through the application of a negative pressure.
- Prefilter pressure, catheter return pressure, and UF port pressure are used in software calculation of transmembrane pressure (TMP), which indicates the capacity of the filter ultrafiltering blood.

- This amount of information, integrated with a friendly, user/operator interface, is optimized in different monitors with different setups and displays. In our opinion, the optimal machine keeps record of circuit pressures during the past 24 treatment hours (or more), and possibly provides graphs and trends of all recorded pressures, and a "log file" of alarms or errors and when they occurred, along with the remedy or operator response at the time. This information is a useful audit of the system in use.

Alarm Systems

Understanding how alarms systems work on CRRT machines is useful for troubleshooting. In general, alarms used in biomedical equipment are classified according to severity of problem and urgency for attention. They range from "advisory" messages, with no immediate error, to "crisis," indicating danger and automatic shutdown. In addition, alarms can be "latched": if a measured parameter is breached, despite self-correction, the machine pauses operation with the alarm sounding until the it is reset. Or, the alarm can be "unlatched": if a breached parameter creates an alarm but the situation self-corrects, the alarm stops and the machine restarts automatically. For example with CRRT machine technology, the low arterial pressure alarm is an unlatched alarm, but an air detection alarm is latched, which represents the potential severity of each alarm. Most new machines provide default settings for many alarms, and sometimes they can be customized. It is useful for staff to know the default settings or the policy in the ICU for when common alarms are set. Alarms set too widely create unsafe use of the machine. Figure 16.1 outlines this concept of alarm classification.

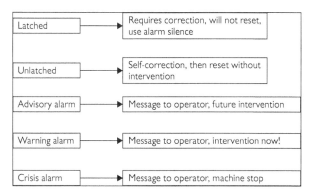

Figure 16.1 Biomedical devices and alarms classification.

The Clogged Circuit

All circuits clot sooner or later, and they generally need the change of all components of the extracorporeal circuit. The first issue to address to optimize management of circuit clotting is prevention. Performing an "elective" change, before the circuit clots completely, allows the reinfusion of circuit blood, preventing secondary anemia. A scheduled change to a new extracorporeal circuit also may allow a reduced time off therapy (downtime).

Some "signs" are indicative of circuit clotting:

- Dark streaks through the hollow fibers of filters indicate a degree of filter clotting proportional to the total amount of clotted fibers. This sign should be kept under constant observation but does not herald imminent filter failure.
- A rapid TMP increase (before it reaches machine alarm threshold) is an important sign of hollow fiber failure, especially during hemofiltration/UF. There is not an absolute value of which to be aware, but more than 250 mmHg is commonly considered indicative of substantial membrane clotting; however, this also depends on machine setup and filter size. The trend curve of TMP should be observed by the operators; if a rapid increase occurs during a short time, a threshold of membrane surface area clotting may be reached and total failure is imminent.
- A rapid DP increase (before it reaches machine alarm threshold) is another important sign of filter clotting and it works as a reliable indicator either during dialysis or hemofiltration/UF. Again, there is not an absolute value of which to be aware (it generally depends on machine setup and filter size). The DP trend curve should be monitored by operators.
- Experience should show the ICU staff that different components in different machines are particularly susceptible to early clotting and should be monitored closely.
- The venous drip chamber (bubble trap) may be a common site of circuit clotting during continuous runs. Two mechanisms seem to be responsible for clot formation: the blood–air interface and blood stagnation in the chamber. Modifications of these chambers, derived from traditional intermittent therapies, have been designed, and new de-aeration chambers without air–blood contact are now available. Keeping the chamber full with a small air space and stopping foaming or splashing of blood flow may also prevent clotting.

Management of Clogged Circuits

Treatment failure resulting from circuit clotting has been acknowledged as the major problem in CRRT delivery. Some general measures are recommended to increase filter life and to achieve an average session length of at least 20 hours:

- Blood flow should, ideally, be prescribed and maintained between 150 mL/min and 200 mL/min. If poor vascular access does not allow this flow rate, and blood flow has to be decreased down to about 100 mL/min the risk of premature clotting is highly increased.
- Administering replacement fluids before the filter may prolong filter function. Alternatively, if postdilution hemofiltration is the preferred institutional CRRT modality, when TMP is increasing rapidly, a switch to predilution hemofiltration, hemodialysis, or hemodiafiltration can be tried (if the machine allows such intratherapy changes).
- If heparin is the administered anticoagulant, the infusion of dilute solutions (10 IU/mL) at a greater rate will improve the efficacy of anticoagulation. In these patients, antithrombin III levels should be monitored, and maintained at supernormal levels (>100%). Activated clotting time or other methods of bedside anticoagulation measures are strongly recommended and, if necessary, the administration of small heparin boluses may be indicated.
- Flushing circuits with normal saline once per shift or when clogging is suspected may allow better visual detection of clot formation in the circuit and sometimes small decreases in circuit pressure. However, the routine flushing of the circuits is not recommended in all cases because of limited efficacy and the fluid administered to patients when doing this frequently.

Troubleshooting for specific events, however, must be decided in the moment. The rapidity of intervention is based on adequate staff training, optimal material choice, and correct CRRT machine setup and/or therapy prescription. Quick interventions reduce circuit failure and downtime, increase system accuracy, and, especially, prevent prolonged cessation or slowing of blood flow, which is the most common cause of clotting.

Fluid Balance Errors

The possibility of making fluid balance errors during CRRT has been identified since the beginning of this modality of treatment. The advent of automated machines has overcome this problem in part. Nevertheless, there are conditions and operation modes in which the potential for fluid balance errors still remain. The precision of delivery of the prescribed renal replacement therapy is dependent on the training of the operators, the clarity of the orders, and the operator's familiarity with the equipment and its fluid measurement accuracy.

Third-generation machines control fluid flows by accurate pump–scales feedback; 30 g (30 mL)/h is the accepted error for each pump, and an alarm warns the operator if this limit is exceeded. Furthermore, some monitors are designed to correct a previous error within the next 60 minutes, increasing the accuracy of the system even further. When therapy is interrupted by a pressure alarm, the machine restarts automatically if the pressure level normalizes within few seconds.

Improvements in commercial machines for safety and accuracy of fluid balance, the way alarms can be overridden, or the occasional addition of external components to the overall fluid balance can easily affect the final result and make fluid balance significantly different from that prescribed. In particular, users who override scale alarms without solving the cause of the alarm (possible error in fluid balance typically occurs when a replacement fluid bag is clamped) may affect patient fluid balance dramatically. In fact, if an alarm appears on the machine, one can override it without major problems: however, after multiple override commands are operated without identifying the problem and solving it adequately the treatment may have inadvertently removed or added a significant amount of fluid to the patient. For this reason, some monitors, by default, accept a limited number of overrides per hour and stop the therapy automatically if the limit is exceeded.

In general, fluid balance errors can be avoided easily not only by correct and careful adherence to the protocols of use of current CRRT machines, but also by compliance with prescriptions and programmed controls during therapy.

Potential fluid balance errors not detected by the machine or errors resulting from inadvertent prescription of additional fluids (diluted drugs, nutrition increase, need for high volumes of blood derivates) should be always considered:

- Physical assessment of the patient and hemodynamic monitor should be constant (especially when CRRT is delivered in semi-intensive care (high-dependency units).
- A fluid balance chart should be updated hourly to interpret patients' total fluid balance correctly.
- Operators should check and possibly record machine information on "effectively delivered net UF" and not just report on the clinical chart the "prescribed net UF.": actual net UF may significantly differ from initially prescribed net UF, as a result of repeated small errors made by the machine (during the 24 hours), but also being caused by all unreported interruptions needed for troubleshooting.

Final Remarks

With any healthcare technology, it is easy to focus on management of the machinery and lose sight of the patient. Therefore, it is invaluable always to have a problem-oriented approach to patients. Constant technical training and checklists are useful for all users and are considered mandatory for novice practitioners (Box 16.1).

Box 16.1 **Troubleshooting Checklist**

It should be noted that modern CRRT machines include, for each alarm that occurs during treatment, an online "real-time" alarm page with clear and simple explanations that describes the causes and remedies for alarms. This alarm page is very useful to operators, but is rarely read and used as a learning tool as a result of the hurry and perceived urgency of the event.

Alarm/ Problem	Possible Cause	Action
Too-low arterial pressure alarm	1. Kinked or clamped line 2. Clotted line 3. Access device against vessel wall 4. Hypovolemia	1. Remove kinking. 2. Declot access. 3. Consider switching limbs. 4. Stop ultrafiltration and decrease blood flow rate
High venous pressure alarm	1. Kinked or clamped line 2. Clotted line 3. Positional vascular access obstruction	1. Remove kinking. 2. Declot access. 3. Consider switching limbs
Arterial (or venous) line disconnection alarm	1. Line separation or disconnection from patient (very rare!) 2. Circuit kinked or clamped before pressure sensor 3. Clot excluding pressure sensor 4. Blood pump speed relatively too slow with respect to catheter performance	1. Check circuit and patient and, if no disconnection is present, override alarm. 2. Declamp line. 3. Evaluate for circuit change. 4. Increase set blood flow rate.
Increasing transmembrane pressure	1. Clogging filter 2. Kinked or clamped dialysis line 3. Blood flow too slow for ultrafiltration setting	1. Evaluate for circuit change. 2. Declamp line. 3. Increase blood flow speed; check ultrafiltration setting,

Box 16.1 Continued

Air in the circuit	1. Presence of small air bubbles (often the result of bicarbonate—CO_2—coming from replacement bags) 2. Line disconnection at arterial access 3. Turbulence close to air sensor	1. Follow instructions for degassing. 2. Stop session. 3. Override alarm.
Fluid balance error	1. Effluent or replacement/dialysis bags moving or hung incorrectly 2. Kinking in effluent or replacement/dialysis bags 3. Machine occasional error 4. Machine systematic error (if more than 10 times without reason in 3 hours).	1. Wait for bags to stop or place them on scales again. 2. Remove line kinking. 3. Override. 4. Change machine and do not reuse it technical assistance is provided.

Key References

Baldwin I. Training, management and credentialing for CRRT in critical care. *Am J Kidney Dis.* 1997;30:S112–S116.

Bellomo R, Baldwin I, Ronco C, Golper T. *Atlas of Hemofiltration.* WB Saunders, Harcourt; 2002.

Parienti JJ, Thirion M, Mégarbane B, Members of the Cathedia Study Group. Femoral vs jugular venous catheterization and risk of nosocomial events in adults requiring acute renal replacement therapy: a randomized controlled trial. *JAMA.* 2008;299:2413–2422.

Ricci Z, Bonello M, Salvatori G, et al. Continuous renal replacement technology: from adaptive technology and early dedicated machines towards flexible multipurpose machine platforms. *Blood Purif.* 2004;22:269–276.

Ronco C, Bellomo R. *Critical Care Nephrology.* 1st ed. Kluwer Academic Publishers, 1998.

Ronco C, Ricci Z, Bellomo R, Baldwin I, Kellum J. Management of fluid balance in CRRT: a technical approach. *Int J Artif Organs.* 2005;28:765–776.

Ronco C, Bellomo R, Kellum JA. *Acute Kidney Injury: Contributions to Nephrology.* Karger Publishers; 2007.

Ronco C, Bellomo R, La Greca G. *Blood Purification in Intensive Care: Contributions to Nephrology.* Karger Publishers; 2002.

www.adqi.org

Chapter 17

Nonanticoagulation Strategies to Optimize Circuit Function in RRT

Ian Baldwin

Key areas for maintaining blood flow and reducing circuit clotting are as follows:

- *Circuit preparation*: Use saline or crystalloid solution to expel all air, avoid excessive tapping to remove air bubbles. Use of bicarbonate fluids for priming may increase bubbles. Addition of heparin during preparation may prevent clotting by coating plastic and membrane surfaces.
- *Access catheter type and site*: Large size, 13.5 to 15.0 For, side-by-side lumen configuration (Figure 17.1). Insertion of the catheter forfor tip placement close to the right atrium on chest radiograph. A femoral site functions well in most patients and is lower risk for clinicians unskilled in insertion. Test access patency by aspiration, and flush at each circuit connection. Access failure resulting from kinking or tissue occlusion can cause reduced blood flow, with pump failure resulting from inadequate pump tubing segment refill (Figure 17.2). If subtle, arterial pressure will be excessive (exceeding negative 100 mmHg). An operator may be unaware this is occurring unless an alarm sounds; premature clotting is the result.
- For *blood flow rate setting*:the optimal setting is 150 to 200 mL/min. Flow must be adequate for the ultrafiltration rate as slow blood flow with high fluid removal causes haemoconcentration and possible clotting. An incorrect blood flow-to-ultrafiltration rate ratio (filtration fraction) causes membrane hemoconcentration, with an increase in clotting and cell clogging of the membrane. A flow that is too fast can cause turbulence at resistance points, cell and plasma separation, and clot formation. A flow that is too slow causes cell slugging and adherence to surfaces.
- *Membrane size and type*: The membrane needs to be adequate for the blood flow and ultrafiltration flow settings. For adults, 1.0 to 1.4 M^2 is appropriate. Different membrane compositions may affect clot potential. When clotting occurs frequently with one type of membrane, try an alternative membrane.
- *Replacement fluids administration site*: Replacement fluids given before the membrane dilute the blood and reduce clot development in the membrane (predilution) (Figure 17.3).

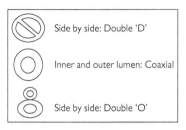

Figure 17.1 Vascular access catheter design profiles.

- *Understanding the "air-bubble trap" chamber*: The bubble trap collects air that enters the circuit before blood returns to the patient. CO_2 bubbles also contribute to this and occur frequently when using heated bicarbonate solutions. The gas and blood interface, along with surface movement, causes cell smearing on the chamber walls. Adjustment of the blood level high in the chamber may reduce cell smearing by reducing the amount of blood splashing on the surface (Figure 17.4). Administering Postdilution fluids into the chamber can create a fluid layer on top of the blood level, possibly reducing clot development (Figure 17.5).

- *Training and education for staff*: Staff training and education have a direct relationship to success and, therefore, circuit life. Machine alarm troubleshooting, recognition of access failure, and use of anticoagulation are key areas for education and training.

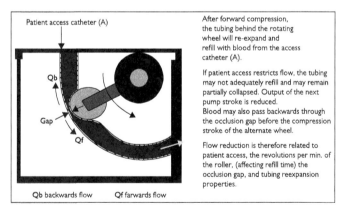

Figure 17.2 Roller pumps: Schematic showing the compression of pump tubing to achieve forward blood flow (Qf) and with access catheter failure backwads flow occurs (Qb).

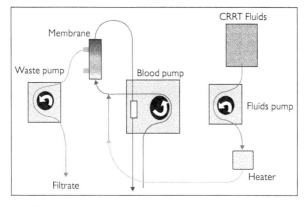

Figure 17.3 Continuous venovenous hemodialysis (CVVH) predilution.

Key ideas for preventing circuit clotting

Clotting in the circuit during continuous renal replacement therapy can be prevented by paying attention to circuit preparation, with air-bubble removal and addition of heparin into the circuit with priming, and circuit connection to a large French vascular access catheter with side-by-side lumen design. Reliable

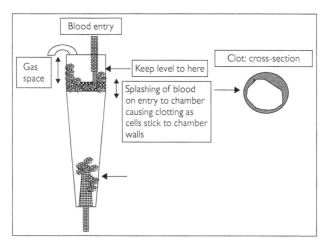

Figure 17.4 Schematic for a bubble trap in the CRRT circuit indicating how clotting develops inside due to splashing and surface rise and fall during use.

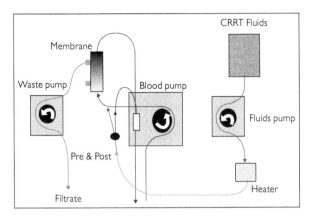

Figure 17.5 Continuors venovenous hemodialysis (CVVH) with pre and post dilution.

and uninterrupted blood flow is essential to prevent stasis and clotting, use of a larger surface area membrane in adults, premembrane substitution fluids administration, and keeping the blood level in the venous bubble trap high, and providing postdilution fluid administration. Nursing training and troubleshooting ability is also vital to prevent clotting resulting from delayed alarm correction and aims for skilled use of this technology in the ICU.

Key References

Baldwin I. Training management and credentialing for CRRT in critical care. *Am J Kidney Dis*. 1997; 30(5):S112–S116.

Baldwin I, Bellomo R. The relationship between blood flow, access catheter and circuit failure during CRRT: a practical review. *Contrib Nephrol*. 2004;144:203–213.

Baldwin I, Bellomo R, Koch W. Blood flow reductions during continuous renal replacement therapy and circuit life. *Intensive Care Med*. 2004;30:2074–2079.

Baldwin I, Tan HK, Bridge N, Bellomo R. Possible strategies to prolong circuit life during hemofiltration: three controlled studies. *Renal Fail*. 2002;24(6):839–848.

Boyle M, Baldwin I. Understanding the continuous renal replacement therapy circuit for acute renal failure support: a quality issue in the intensive care unit. *AACN*. 2010;21(4):365–375.

Canaud B, Formet C, Raynal N, et al. Vascular access for extracorporeal renal replacement therapy in the intensive care unit. *Contrib Nephrol*. 2004;144:291–307.

Egi M, Naka T, Bellomo R, et al. A comparison of two citrate anticoagulation regimens for continuous veno-venous hemofiltration. *J Artif Organs*. 2005;28(12):1211–1218.

Lavaud S, Paris B, Maheut H, et al. Assessment of the heparin-binding AN69 ST hemodialysis membrane: II. Clinical studies without heparin administration. *ASAIO J*. 2005;51(4):348–351.

Oudemans-Van Straaten HM, Wester JPJ, de Pont ACJM, Schetz MRC. Anticoagulation strategies in continuous renal replacement therapy: can the choice be evidence based? *Intensive Care Med.* 2006;32:188–202.

Tolwani AJ, Wille K. Anticoagulation for continuous renal replacement therapy. *Semin Dialysis.* 2009;22(2):141–145.

Uchino S, Fealy N, Baldwin I, Morimatsu H, Bellomo R. Pre-dilution vs. post-dilution during continuous veno-venous hemofiltration: impact on filter life and azotemic control. *Nephron Clin Pract.* 2003;94(4):94–98.

Webb AR, Mythen MG, Jacobsen D, Mackie IJ. Maintaining blood flow in the extracorporeal circuit: haemostasis and anticoagulation. *Intensive Care Med.* 1995;21:84–93.

Chapter 18

Anticoagulation

Rinaldo Bellomo and Ian Baldwin

Introduction

Continuous treatment suggests extracorporeal blood flow without clotting, which is not a realistic aim. However, drugs that block normal coagulation pathways can prevent or delay clotting such that sufficient treatment time is achieved and, more important, patient blood is returned before complete circuit obstruction. Anticoagulation refers primarily to the use of agents that prevent blood from clotting after contact with the plastic and artificial surfaces in the extracorporeal circuit. Heparin is used most commonly as an anticoagulant for renal replacement therapy by blocking factor Xa and thrombin. Citrate is also used routinely to prevent clotting by chelating calcium and by preventing its action as a cofactor. Administration of anticoagulant drugs during renal replacement therapy requires specific knowledge and the application of monitoring protocols to ensure safety and effectiveness. This chapter provides a brief clinical guide to such treatment.

The following is a list of Key Areas for Attention When Administering an Anticoagulant for the Prevention of Circuit Clotting

- Develop a bedside protocol for anticoagulant use. Keep it simple and readily available for reference as a chart or computer page.
- Develop your own expertise with this protocol.
- If the circuit clots, it can be replaced. If the patient bleeds, a more serious and adverse outcome may occur. To lose a filter to protect a patient is entirely acceptable. To lose a patient to protect a filter is not.
- Often, the circuit clots not because anticoagulation is suboptimal or inadequate, but rather because of poor-quality vascular access, poor attention to optimal machine operation, and sudden changes in patient position that alter catheter function, decrease blood flow, and induce clotting through stasis. To respond to such events by increasing the anticoagulant dose is

dangerous and unwise. For every clotting event, an appropriate diagnostic assessment is necessary to implement rational measures to prevent it the next time around.

The following is a list of Practical Considerations Using Heparin Anticoagulation

- It is not necessary to use full heparin anticoagulation to perform continuous renal replacement therapy (CRRT). Many patients have low platelet counts and altered clotting as a result of critical illness.
- After major surgery and with epidural use, no anticoagulation for the first 24 to 48 hours postoperatively, or citrate anticoagulation, maybe a safer option.
- CRRT machines include a syringe device for concentrated anticoagulant drug preparation. If a dilute preparation is used, an intravenous pump used widely in the ward promotes safety because all staff should be familiar with its operation.
- Use of dilute preparation administered by volumetric pump minimizes accidental bolus and syringe "lag" when changing the syringe after it is empty.
- Make the heparin infusion preparation simple in terms of calculation of dose. This strategy makes orders and communication easier and safer. Heparin at 10,000 IU in a 1000-mL bag = 10 IU/mL.
- Label and identify this infusion as FOR CRRT ONLY.
- Use a heparin preparation different from those used for other anticoagulation prescriptions (e.g., after thrombosis or embolism).
- Use a dosing chart or table (Table 18.1) based on body weight for initial heparin bolus dose and consideration of the daily clotting profile for the patient.
- Adding heparin to the priming solution may provide some benefit to stop clotting, but this strategy is not proved.

Table 18.1 Heparin dosing guide for bolus and infusion			
Heparin Infusion Rate	INR	APTT	Platelets
10 IU/kg/h	<1.5	<40 s	>150 x 10^9/mL
5 IU/kg/h	>15 but <2.5	>40 s but <60 s	<150 x 10^9/mL but >75 x 10^9/mL
No bolus, no anticoagulation	>2.5	>60 s	<75 x 10^9/mL

Activated Partial Thromboplastin Time, APTT; International Normalised Ratio, INR. All circuits to have a 5000-IU bolus of heparin if infusion is planned. Thereafter adjust heparin according to the principles outlined in the table. If one of the criteria for coagulation is present, adjust the dosage accordingly.

- Start the treatment using the dosing table as a guide, then increase heparin if circuit life is poor. If filter life is less than 8 hours for the first circuit, consider increasing the dosage. A filter life of 20 to 24 hours is common using heparin correctly and this method is "working." A dosage of 5 to 10 IU/kg/h given prefilter is a common starting dosage for the first treatment circuit.
- The fluid volume used to administer the anticoagulant must be included in the fluid balance calculations (i.e., is added to the loss setting).
- Administering the anticoagulant into the circuit before blood enters the membrane in the "prefilter" position is common and makes sense.
- Check and assess the patient for evidence of spontaneous bleeding. Also monitor the urine, feces, wounds, punctures sites, and mucus membranes for blood .
- Do not check the patient clotting time Activate Partial Thromboplastin Time (APTT) too frequently and make inappropriate infusion adjustments. Check after the first 6 hours. After that, 12-hour monitoring is probably adequate in most cases unless significant clinical changes have taken place. After stabilization, daily monitoring is adequate. If patient anticoagulation is the goal, APTT monitoring may need to be more frequent. If circuit antico-agulation is the goal, APTT monitoring is performed, not to titrate heparin infusion, but rather to ensure there is no unnecessary or excessive patient anticoagulation.
- Have a simple table to explain less common approaches to anticoagulation for the nursing staff (Table 18.2)
- Chart the dose of heparin given each hour on bedside observation charts/ computers and the filter consecutive hours of function next to this value. This strategy provides an instant ability to assess filter life associated with heparin dosing (Table 18.3).

Summary of key issues when using anticoagulants for CRRT

Anticoagulants can delay or prevent circuit clotting. However, they increase the risk of bleeding. Therefore, their use should be based on a careful assessment of the likely risks and benefits in a given patient. Heparin is used commonly in hospitals. Typically, doctors and nurses understand its risks and benefits well, and have established expertise with this drug. Heparin, however, is not always necessary, and CRRT can be done without its use, particularly in patients at high risk of bleeding (low platelet count, a prolonged International Normalised Ratio INR, and prolonged APTT). Heparin can be reversed with protamine if necessary. Use of a standard dilute preparation, administration prefilter via a common infusion device, reference to a dosing chart specific for CRRT, and ongoing review of patients and their clotting profile all promote safe circuit anticoagulation. No other approaches to circuit anticoagulation have yet been

Table 18.2 Outline of less common approaches to circuit anticoagulation

Drug	Infusion	Where?	Comment
Regional heparin/ protamine	Protamine at 10 mg/ h and heparin at 1000 units/h (1:100 ratio)	Heparin is administered prefilter and protamine is administered postfilter into the venous chamber or directly into the return limb of the access catheter via a suitable Y piece (not a three-way tap).	Not with HIT. Check patient APTT after 6 hours to ensure that heparin effect is reversed.
PGI2	Bolus (5 ng/kg/ min) over 15 minutes before commencement of CRRT via a CVC; infusion, 4–8 ng/ kg/min	Circuit prefilter	Hypotension, bleeding. and/or abdominal cramps may occur with PGI2 therapy.
Danaparoid	Bolus of 750 IU/h, 1–2 IU/kg/h	Circuit prefilter	Check daily anti-Xa level of 0.2–0.35 IU/mL.

Activated Partial Thromboplastin Time, (APTT); CRRT, continuous renal replacement therapy, Central Venous Catheter (CVC), Heparin Induced Thrombocytopaenia (HIT), Prostaglandin (PGI2) or Epoprostenol/prostacyclin.

shown to be superior to heparin, although citrate anticoagulation is also highly effective and emerging as a first preference. Whatever the choice of approach to anticoagulation, physicians and nurses must remain vigilant for changes in the patient's risk profile, and make a frequent and thoughtful assessment of which approach to circuit anticoagulation is best at any given time in a given patient.

Table 18.3 Intensive care unit charting approach that aligns hourly vital signs observations with heparin dose each hour with accompanying filter "life"

Heparin Dose IU /hr	500	500	500	500		750	750
Filter Hour	7	8	9	10	Clotted	1	2

Key References

Fealy N, Baldwin I, Johnstone M, Egi M, Bellomo R. A pilot controlled crossover study comparing regional heparinization to regional citrate anticoagulation for continuous venovenous hemofiltration. *Int J Artif Organs*. 2007;30:281–292.

Joannidis M, Oudemans-van Straaten HM. Clinical review: patency of the circuit in continuous renal replacement therapy. *Crit Care*. 2007;11(4):218.

Naka T, Egi M, Bellomo R, et al. Commercial low-citrate anticoagulation haemofiltration in high risk patients with frequent filter clotting. *Anaesth Intensive Care*. 2005;33:601–608.

Oudemans-van Straaten HM, Kellum JA, Bellomo R. Clinical review: anticoagulation for continuous renal replacement therapy: heparin or citrate? *Crit Care*. 2011:15:202–210.

Tan HK, Baldwin I, Bellomo R. Hemofiltration without anticoagulation in high-risk patients. *Intensive Care Med*. 2000;26:1652–1657.

Uchino S, Fealy N, Baldwin I, Morimatsu H, Bellomo R. Continuous hemofiltration without anticoagulation. *ASAIO J*. 2004;50:76–80.

Chapter 19

Regional Citrate Anticoagulation

Nigel Fealy

Method

It is important to understand some aspects of calcium physiology and distribution in blood (Figure 19.1). When citrate is infused into the blood circuit, it combines with ionized calcium to form citrate–calcium complexes (nonionized), which reduce the level of ionized calcium in the extracorporeal circuit and in turn leads to the inhibition of clotting in the circuit. The target for the *circuit* ionized serum calcium level to prevent or retard clotting is generally between 0.25 mmol/L and 0.4 mmol/L.

There is no systemic anticoagulation as a result of the following:

- There is significant loss of the citrate–calcium complexes as they cross the semipermeable membrane of the filter into the effluent.
- Any citrate or citrate–calcium complexes that remain in the venous line and are delivered to the patient are diluted with the patient's blood and are metabolized rapidly by liver, kidney, and muscle cells to form free bicarbonate (one citrate ion = three bicarbonate ions).
- During this metabolism of the citrate–calcium complexes, calcium liberated from the complex contributes to the normalization of calcium levels.
- Serum ionized calcium levels lost in the waste are replaced by the administration of a calcium infusion to the patient, restoring normal levels (normal serum ionized calcium level, ~1.1–1.3 mmol/L).

A variety of citrate protocols or regimens exist for continuous renal replacement therapy (CRRT) with a major difference in approach between continuous venovenous hemofiltration (CVVH) and continuous venovenous hemodiafiltration (CVVHDF) as therapy. Often, protocols are hospital or intensive care unit specific, requiring pharmacy or custom-made solutions (substitution and dialysate) to implement the technique. These prescriptions vary according to mode, pre- or postdilution, different citrate solutions, different approaches for monitoring, and adjusting for acid–base control.

In CRRT, there are three major forms of citrate used. One is 4% trisodium citrate, another is acid citrate dextrose solution, and a third is citrate containing

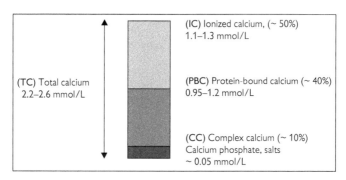

Figure 19.1 Calcium distribution in plasma and normal lab ranges.

replacement solutions. These different approaches vary primarily for mode of CRRT, such as a pure diffusive method (continuous venovenous hemodialysis), a diffusive and convective method (CVVHDF), and a pure convective method (CVVH). A description of protocols for CVVHDF and CVVH are illustrated in Figure 19.2 and Figure 19.3, respectively.

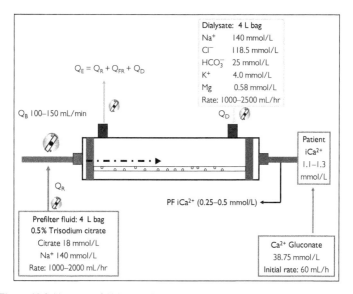

Figure 19.2 University of Alabama at Birmingham continuous venovenous hemodiafiltration protocol. *Source:* Tolwani A, Prendergast M, Speer R, Stofan B, Willie K. A practical citrate anticoagulation continuous venovenous hemodiafiltration protocol for metabolic control and high solute clearance. *Clin J Am Soc Nephrol.* 2005;1:79–87.

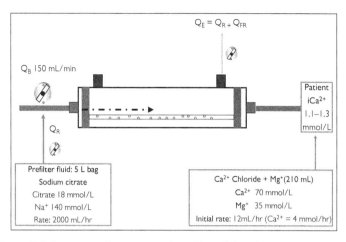

Figure 19.3 Department of intensive care, Austin Hospital, Australia, continuous venovenous hemofiltration protocol. Q_B, blood flow; Q_E, effluent flow; Q_{FR}, fluid removal; Q_R, replacement.

Practical Considerations

Key considerations for maintaining metabolic and electrolyte balance are as follows:

- In addition to providing an anticoagulant, citrate acts as an acid buffer after liver metabolism. One millimole of citrate yields 3 mmol bicarbonate when metabolized. Potentially, when higher doses of citrate are administered, this could lead to an increase in serum bicarbonate levels (metabolic alkalosis).
- The amount of citrate lost in CRRT waste or ultrafiltrate varies with ultrafiltrate flow rate (both ultrafiltration rate and amount of fluid removal), and therefore the amount of buffer entering the systemic circulation may vary or may be inadequate (metabolic acidosis).
- When trisodium citrate is used, there is an increase in sodium load to the patient, increasing the risk of hypernatremia.
- If the patient is not able to metabolize citrate–calcium complexes as a result of liver dysfunction or via the skeletal muscle pathway, then citrate may accumulate and no buffer is generated. In addition hypocalcemia may also result.
- In addition to binding calcium to form calcium–citrate complexes, magnesium is also bound and filters freely across the membrane, potentially leading to a reduction in serum magnesium levels.

When prescribing a citrate-based anticoagulation regimen, metabolic monitoring should be a priority. Regular monitoring of pH, serum, and circuit ionized calcium, serum bicarbonate, sodium, and magnesium levels should be an essential element of any unit-based protocol. Depending on the method used, a local protocol should be developed to monitor, report, and treat any metabolic derangements that may occur as a result of using a citrate-based anticoagulation regimen. There are numerous descriptions and reports available for the monitoring of electrolytes, acid–base balance, and anticoagulation in regional citrate anticoagulation (RCA).

Efficacy and safety of RCA

RCA has shown to be significantly more efficient in maintaining patency of the CRRT circuit compared to other anticoagulation strategies including unfractionated heparin. The major advantage is that superior anticoagulation can be achieved for CRRT without the need for systemic anticoagulation and risk of bleeding in critically ill patients. The choice of citrate protocol depends largely on the citrate solution available, mode of therapy used (CVVH, CVVHDF), and method chosen for citrate delivery (infusion as a concentrate or additive to a replacement solution). RCA requires unit-based protocols that are easy to follow, provide safety as a priority, and are practical in design. Recent technological advances have allowed the introduction of these protocols into specific software on many commercially available CRRT machines. These systems allow automated adjustments of blood flow rate, citrate dose, calcium replacement and ultrafiltrate dose . With these protocols and improved machine software in place, RCA is a safe and effective strategy for anticoagulation in CRRT.

Key References

Abramson S, Niles J. Anticoagulation for continuous renal replacement therapy. *Curr Opin Nephrol Hypertens*. 1999;8:701–707.

Cointault O, Kamar N, Bories P, et al. Regional citrate anticoagulation in continuous venovenous haemodiafiltration using commercial solutions. *Nephrol Dial Transplant*. 2003;19(1):171–178.

Davies H, Morgan D, Leslie G. A regional citrate anticoagulation protocol for pre-dilution CVVHDF: the "modified Alabama Protocol." *Austr Crit Care*. 2009;21(3):154–165.

Fealy N, Baldwin I, Johnstone MJ, Egi M, Bellomo R. A pilot randomized controlled crossover study comparing regional heparinization to regional citrate anticoagulation for continuous venovenous hemofiltration. *Int J Artif Organs*. 2007;30(4):301–307.

Kutsogiannis DJ, Mayers I, Chin W, Gibney R. Regional citrate anticoagulation in continuous venovenous hemofiltration. *Am J Kidney Dis*. 2000;35:802–811.

Tolwani A, Prendergast M, Speer R, Stofan B, Willie K. A practical citrate anticoagulation continuous venovenous hemodiafiltration protocol for metabolic control and high solute clearance. *Clin J Am Soc Nephrol.* 2005;1:79–87.

Tolwani A, Wille K. Anticoagulation for continuous renal replacement therapy. *Semin Dial.* 2009;22(2):141–145.

Gattas DJ, Bradford C, Rajbhandari D, Buhr H, Lo S, Bellomo R. A randomized controlled trial of regional citrate versusregional heparin anticoagulation for continuous renal replacement therapy in critically ill adults. Critical Care Medicine. 2015, 43(8):1622-9

Stucker F, Ponte B, Tataw J, Martin PY, Wozniak H, Pugin J, Saudan P. Efficacy and safety of citrate-based anticoagulation compared to heparin in patients with acute kidney injury requiring continuous renal replacement therapy: a randomized controlled trial. Critical Care. 2015, 19:91

Chapter 20

Drug Dosing in Continuous Renal Replacement Therapy

Adrian Wong, Sandra L. Kane-Gill, and John A. Kellum

Acute kidney injury (AKI) in the intensive care unit (ICU) occurs in 5% to 25% of patients. Of this population, approximately 6% require renal replacement therapy (RRT). Mortality in patients requiring RRT is estimated to be even higher than in patients with AKI not requiring RRT (60%), approaching up to 80%.

Modes of RRT include intermittent hemodialysis (IHD) or continuous renal replacement therapy (CRRT). CRRT offers the potential advantage of continuous removal of fluid and solutes, reducing potential fluctuations in electrolytes, fluid balance, and hemodynamic stability, compared with IHD. Although there is ongoing debate regarding the optimal use and application of RRT in the ICU, its frequent use necessitates drug dosing considerations. Along with the numerous comorbidities and physiological factors that may affect drug dosing in critically ill patients, RRT only adds to the complicated nature of these patients.

Numerous variables affect drug dosing in patients receiving RRT, including mode of RRT, pharmacokinetic and pharmacodynamic (PD) changes in the critically ill patient, and physiochemical properties that affect drug dosing and clearance. These variables further complicate the importance of appropriate dosing of drugs to maximize patient outcome and minimize potential patient harm. A contributing factor to the high mortality rate in ICU patients receiving RRT could be the mismanagement of antibiotic dosing from accelerated drug clearance during RRT, especially with the higher doses of CRRT currently used. Although "renal impairment" studies are completed during drug development per the Food and Drug Administration, quality data regarding the proper dosing of drugs in RRT and especially CRRT are currently lacking. This lack of data leads to significant practice variation. Although this chapter focuses on antibiotic dosing, given its importance and prevalence in ICU patients, the strategies for dosing may be applied to other drugs as well.

CRRT Properties

As discussed in Chapters 10 and 12, CRRT can be applied using various techniques and methods. Differences among CRRT techniques affecting clearance include mechanism of solute clearance, type of vascular access, filter membrane properties, and flow rates for blood, ultrafiltration, and dialysis fluid.

CRRT Techniques

The three main techniques of clearance used are hemodialysis, hemofiltration, and hemodiafiltration. Each technique varies in mechanism of solute clearance, need for fluid replacement, and amount of solute clearance (Table 20.1). In addition, each technique can be applied using either arteriovenous or venovenous access. Venovenous methods are generally preferred, given the reduced risk of complications and the ability to generate consistent and higher solute clearance rates. The following describes various differences between clearance techniques.

- *Hemodialysis* uses passive diffusion of solutes across a concentration gradient with countercurrent dialysis fluid. Only molecules of small molecular weight (<500 Da) are readily removed during diffusion. Replacement fluid is not required.
- *Hemofiltration* uses convection, during which solutes and plasma water are driven through a membrane with a pressure gradient, resulting in higher solute removal and the formation of an ultrafiltrate. As long as the solute is smaller than the pore size cutoff for the membrane used, particle size or molecular weight have little influence on solute removal during convection methods. However, replacement fluid, which can be administered before or after blood ultrafiltration, is required because of the large volume of ultrafiltrate formed during this process.
- *Hemodiafiltration* is a combination of diffusion and convection. Solute and volume removal involve a countercurrent dialysis fluid and pressure gradient. Replacement fluids are required to support higher ultrafiltration rates.
- *Slow continuous ultrafiltration (SCUF)* is a therapy of fluid removal without dialysis or replacement fluid. SCUF is not appropriate for patients with renal failure because it provides only very limited solute clearance. SCUF is usually used for temporary volume removal in patients with at least some renal function (e.g., congestive heart failure). As such, drug dosing does not typically require adjustment for patients receiving SCUF.

Table 20.1 Continuous renal replacement therapy techniques			
Technique	**Clearance mechanism**		**Replacement fluid**
	Convection	**Diffusion**	
CVVH	++++	0	+++
CVVHD	+	++++	0
CVVHDF	+++	+++	++
SCUF	+	0	0

0, none; +, minimal; ++, low; +++, medium; ++++, high; CVVH, continuous venovenous hemofiltration; CVVHD, continuous venovenous hemodialysis; CVVHDF, continuous venovenous hemodiafiltration; SCUF, slow continuous ultrafiltration.

In general, overall drug removal may be expected to be greater with CRRT compared with IHD, and when replacement fluids are administered after filtration. Drug clearance is greatest with continuous venovenous hemodiafiltration followed by continuous venovenous hemodialysis, and then continuous venovenous hemofiltration. However, drug clearance with CRRT may vary greatly depending on their particular physicochemical properties, and the CRRT device characteristics and operating conditions.

Filter Properties

Filters used in CRRT differ in a number of properties, including permeability, membrane composition, and surface area. Although no one membrane is recommended, it is important to note their differences and to understand that different filters may result in significant differences in solute or drug removal.

Membrane Permeability

Membrane permeability differs on the basis of the type of RRT used. Conventional low-flux IHD hemodialyzers have smaller pore sizes and are inefficient at removing molecules larger than 500 Da. Conversely, filters that are used in CRRT have increased pore size and are effective in removing molecules up to 50,000 Da. Another factor affecting permeability is the age of the CRRT filter. Solute removal may decrease with an increase in age of the filter, resulting from protein clogging or clotting that occurs over time. In fact, as a result of circuit downtime, patients receive only approximately 70% of their prescribed dose of CRRT, affecting solute clearance, especially when the patient does not have any residual renal function.

The ability of a drug or solute to pass through a filter membrane is expressed as the sieving coefficient (SC). Drugs with an SC that approaches one, are able to pass through the filter freely and require increased drug dosing or decreased time between dosing intervals. The SC is available for some drugs in published literature; otherwise, it can be calculated by obtaining drug concentrations and dividing the ultrafiltration drug concentration by the plasma concentration.

Flow Rates

Although variation exists depending on which mode of therapy and which membranes are used, in general, higher flow rates (blood flow, dialysate flow, ultrafiltration flow) result in increased solute removal. Flow rate has the largest effect of all variables on drug clearance in patients on CRRT. Hence, for drugs removed by CRRT, increased flow rates result in a need to increase drug dosing or to decrease time between dosing intervals. The prescribed total flow rate may be converted from liters per hour to milliliters per minute to provide a rough estimation of renal clearance. For example, a rate of 2 L/h would approximate to a clearance of 30 mL/min. This does not take into account multiple factors, including circuit downtime, modality of CRRT, and drug or patient properties. Therefore, this method serves only as a rough estimation and should not be used when data guiding drug dosing are available.

Patient Properties

Critically ill patients may have alterations in their pharmacokinetic parameters that can affect drug clearance and disposition. With regard to drug dosing in CRRT, relevant patient changes include volume of distribution (Vd), protein binding, metabolism, and elimination:

- *Volume of distribution*: Vd may be altered in critically ill patients, with either an increase or decrease in total body water and intravascular volume. For example, in patients with septic shock, patients initially have a large Vd as a result of cytokine release, which only increases with volume resuscitation. Vd is the largest factor in drug dosing during the initial stages of septic shock and, therefore, loading doses are necessary to obtain therapeutic levels quickly. Therefore, larger doses of drugs with a large Vd are necessary until septic shock resolves or fluid is removed through CRRT. Patients may then require lower doses of drugs as they are brought back to their initial weight. In addition, patients who are obese may require increased doses of drugs to account for an increased Vd, although these data are even more limited given this specific patient population. These doses may approach that of patients who have preserved renal function. The presence of extracorporeal membrane oxygenation may also increase Vd, adding another factor to complicate drug dosing.

- *Protein binding*: Critically ill patients may be affected by several variables, including acid–base disturbances and alterations in protein concentrations. Acid–base abnormalities affect protein binding adversely. Studies performed in the critically ill show that a decrease in the concentration of albumin or an increase in the concentration of alpha-1-acid glycoprotein may occur. Given that only the unbound fraction of a drug is able to diffuse across a filter membrane, shifts in protein concentrations or acid–base status can affect the amount of unbound drug (i.e. active drug) available in the body. These changes can ultimately affect the amount of drug available for removal by CRRT. More important, protein binding is in dynamic equilibrium. Because of its continuous nature, CRRT results in significantly greater removal of drugs with increased protein binding compared with IHD.

- *Metabolism*: Assessment of other organ function is essential to determine the potential for accumulation of metabolites as well as parent compounds. Drug metabolism may be altered in renal failure, leading to altered hepatic metabolism and resulting in altered systemic clearance.

- *Elimination*: The application of CRRT is more likely to increase the clearance of drugs eliminated renally than those that undergo nonrenal clearance mechanisms. Studies have indicated that nonrenal clearance of drugs may increase when AKI initially occurs, but decreases as CRRT is initiated. Nonrenal clearance is dominated by hepatic clearance, but includes other organs as well. Drugs exhibiting altered clearance include imipenem, meropenem, and vancomycin. Alterations to drug elimination include altered cytochrome P450 and P-glycoprotein systems, which may result in the accumulation of active metabolites. Figure 20.1 offers additional information regarding nonrenal clearance. The existence of residual renal function must also be considered as this may further enhance drug clearance in a patient undergoing CRRT. The addition of residual renal function to CRRT clearance should be considered to ensure adequate dosing of drugs, especially antibiotics. Furthermore, fluid removal by CRRT may result in changes in drug elimination by other organs.

- *Other factors*: Other potential factors that may influence drug dosing are detailed in an example with antimicrobials. Dosing may be required to be higher in patients based on the suspected severity of infection, in patients who have an impaired immune system, and in patients with deep-seated infection. In addition, antibiotic dosing may require higher dosing in patients with a hypermetabolic state, including burn injury patients. Finally, transdermal, subcutaneous, and oral administration drug absorption can also be affected significantly by volume overload and by peripheral and intestinal edema. Because edema is reduced with CRRT, enteral drug absorption may increase.

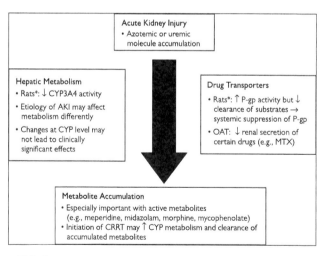

Figure 20.1 Alterations in nonrenal clearance resulting from acute kidney injury. *Rats were induced with AKI primarily via uranyl nitrate. For P-gp, expression was increased in the kidney, but not in the liver or intestines. AKI, acute kidney injury; CRRT, continuous renal replacement therapy; CY, cytochrome; MTX, methotrexate; OAT, organic anion transporter; P-gp, P-glycoprotein.

Drug Properties

There are a number of intrinsic properties that affect the ability of any drug to be removed by CRRT. These properties include molecular weight, protein binding, Vd, and elimination mechanisms.

Molecular Weight

Although the molecular weight of a drug is a consideration, improved technology in regard to size of membrane pores has decreased the importance of this factor significantly.

Protein Binding

The degree to which any drug is bound to protein affects its ability to be cleared by CRRT (Table 20.2). Drugs that are bound to proteins form large complex molecules (>50,000 Da) and are not readily removed by IHD or CRRT. Unbound drugs are more likely to pass through a filter and require increased drug dosing or a decreased time between dosing intervals. A rough estimate of drug clearance may be estimated by multiplying the unbound fraction of the drug by the total flow rate of the CRRT.

Drugs with SCs that are low or near zero cannot be removed by CRRT. Drugs with high protein binding are removed to a small extent only with CRRT and not at all with IHD.

Volume of Distribution

Drugs that have a small Vd are generally hydrophilic and limited to the vascular space because they are unable to pass through plasma membranes. Most hydrophilic agents are eliminated renally as unchanged drug. Therefore, drugs with a low Vd are removed more readily by CRRT and may require increased or more frequent dosing. Examples include aminoglycosides, β-lactams, and glycopeptides, with the exceptions of ceftriaxone, nafcillin, and oxacillin. These drugs undergo primary biliary elimination and therefore are largely unaffected by CRRT despite their hydrophilic status.

Table 20.2 Relative sieving coefficients and protein binding of commonly used drugs

Drug	SC	PB	Drug	SC	PB
Acyclovir	+++	Very low	Digoxin	+++	Low
Amphotericin	+	Very high	Gentamicin	++	Very low
Ampicillin	++	Low	Imipenem	+++	Low
Ceftazidime	+++	Very low	Oxacillin	0	Very high
Ciprofloxacin	++	Low	Phenytoin	+	High
Cyclosporine	++	Very high	Piperacillin	++	Low
Diazepam	0	Very high	Vancomycin	++	Very low

0, approximately 0; +, 0.1-0.5; ++, 0.6-0.8; +++, ≥ 0.9; PB, protein binding; SC, sieving coefficient.

Conversely, lipophilic drugs are able to cross plasma membranes freely and sequester into tissues; they typically have a large Vd and undergo hepatic metabolism. Drugs with a large Vd are less available to pass through the CRRT circuit for clearance and therefore are less affected by renal clearance changes (i.e. extracorporeal or residual). CRRT may have a greater effect on drug removal because the increased duration of therapy increases the likelihood that the drug redistributes from the tissue to vascular space and is available for clearance. Examples include chloramphenicols, fluoroquinolones, macrolides, rifamycins, and tetracyclines, with the exceptions of levofloxacin and ciprofloxacin, which undergo renal elimination and may be removed by CRRT despite their lipophilic nature.

Elimination

Drugs that are cleared renally likely require dosing adjustment during RRT. In addition, dosing requirements may be increased further in patients with residual or recovering renal function receiving CRRT. Patients who are being converted from CRRT to IHD as a result of improving hemodynamic stability should have their drugs preemptively dose-adjusted for the expected decrease in drug elimination. This tactic may minimize potential adverse outcomes, including supratherapeutic levels of drugs, which is especially important in patients with recovering renal function for drugs associated with inducing renal injury, such as acyclovir, aminoglycosides, and β-lactams. Finally, dosing should occur after IHD is performed to maintain adequate serum concentrations.

Pharmacodynamic Principles

Appropriate dosing of antimicrobial agents in patients receiving CRRT is necessary and must include PD considerations. Studies of critically ill patients indicate subtherapeutic levels of drugs, including antibiotics, that may potentially lead to treatment failure, increased antibiotic resistance, and increased mortality. In brief, antimicrobial efficacy has been defined in PD terms to be either concentration-dependent or time-dependent.

Concentration-Dependent Antimicrobials

The efficacy of concentration-dependent antimicrobials is related primarily to the peak serum concentration (C_{max})-to-minimum inhibitory concentration (MIC) ratio (C_{max}/MIC) and the area under the curve (AUC)-to-MIC (AUC/MIC) ratios. Concentration-dependent antimicrobials include aminoglycosides, fluoroquinolones, glycopeptides. and metronidazole. AUC/MIC ratios greater than 100 have been suggested for Gram-negative organisms, and more than 30 for Gram-positive organisms. C_{max}/MIC ratios of 10 to 12 have been shown to provide clinical efficacy and prevent the development of resistance. Concentration-dependent agents exhibit postantibiotic effects against Gram-positive and Gram-negative organisms; therefore, allowing concentrations to fall below the MIC is permissible and may reduce the incidence of adverse effects. Concentration-dependent drugs typically require increased doses to achieve adequate PD parameters.

Time-Dependent Antimicrobials

The efficacy of time-dependent antimicrobials is related primarily to the duration of time the drug concentration exceeds the MIC or by maintaining the minimum plasma concentration (C_{min}) above the MIC. Time-dependent agents include azoles, β-lactams, and oxazolidinones. Maximum efficacy is achieved by maintaining the C_{min} over the MIC for a certain period of time, which is dependent on the specific antimicrobial. Troughs below the MIC must be avoided in time-dependent agents because the majority, with the exception of carbapenems, lack a postantibiotic effect against Gram-negative organisms. Time-dependent drugs require more frequent dosing or the use of PD dosing strategies, including extended-infusion dosing to achieve adequate time above the MIC.

Dosing Recommendations

There are multiple limitations with regard to dosing recommendations for CRRT. Even with the available literature, there are limitations that may affect the application of findings to various institutions. Available data are quite

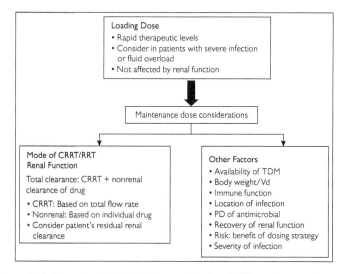

Figure 20.2 Proposed antimicrobial dosing considerations. CRRT, continuous renal replacement therapy; PD, pharmacodynamics; RRT, renal replacement therapy; TDM, therapeutic drug monitoring; Vd, volume of distribution.

heterogenous; variations in the populations and clinical practice at the study institutions may affect the findings in these studies. Study populations vary, and have been identified as including a combination of shock states, such as septic and cardiogenic, which differ in their pathophysiology. Clinical practice variations include modality of CRRT used, basis of dosing of CRRT (flat flow rate vs. weight-based dosing), and the intensity of CRRT. Finally, as the practice of medicine continues to advance, older evidence may not be as applicable to our current patient population resulting from advances in technology affecting

Table 20.3 Selected intravenous antimicrobial maintenance dosing recommendations*

Drug	CVVH	CVVHD	CVVHDF
Acyclovir†	5–10 mg/kg q24h	5-10 mg/kg q12–24h	
Aminoglycosides	Dosing based on levels and adequate to achieve goal C_{max}/MIC: peak for efficacy and trough for safety; goal levels dependent on individual aminoglycoside		
Ampicillin-sulbactam	3 g q12h	3 g q8h	
Aztreonam	1-2 g q12h	2 g q12h	
Cefazolin	1-2 g q12h	2 g q12h	
Cefepime	1–2 g q12h	2 g q12h	
Ceftazidime	1-2 g q12h	2 g q12h	
Ciprofloxacin	200-400 mg q12h	400 mg q12h	
Colistin‡	2.5 mg/kg q48h	Daily dose of CBA to achieve each 1.0 mg/L colistin $C_{ss,avg}$ target = 192 mg with dosing split q8–12h or 160 mg q8h	
Daptomycin	4–6 mg/kg q48h	6–8 mg/kg q48h	
Doripenem	250 mg q8h	250–500 mg q8h	
Fluconazole	200–400 mg q24h	400–800 mg q24h	
Levofloxacin	250 mg q24h	500 mg q24h	750 mg q24h
Meropenem	0.5–1g q12h	0.5–1 g q8–12h	
Piperacillin–tazobactam	2.25–3.375 g q6–8h, 4.5 g q8–12h	2.25–3.375 g q6h, 4.5 g q8h q8–12h	
Piperacillin–tazobactam (extended infusion)	3.375 g q8h, administered over 4 h		
Sulfamethoxazole/trimethoprim§	2.5–7.5 mg/kg q8–12h		
Vancomycin	10–20 mg/kg q24h Alternative: dosing based on vancomycin levels		

CBA, colistin base activity; C_{max}, peak serum concentration; $C_{ss,avg}$, colistin average steady state serum concentration; CVVH, continuous venovenous hemofiltration; CVVHD, continuous venovenous hemodialysis; CVVHDF, continuous venovenous hemodiafiltration; MIC, minimum inhibitory concentration; q, every. *Assume ultrafiltration and dialysis flow rates of 1 to 2 L/h, and minimal residual renal function. †Dosing weight is ideal body weight in obese patients. ‡CBA: 150 mg CBA = 5 MU of colistin methanesulfonate (CMS) = 400 mg CMS sodium. §Dosing based on trimethoprim content.

CRRT removal. Other factors include increasing microbial MICs indicating decreased antimicrobial susceptibility, have continued to change as a result of antibiotic resistance. Figure 20.2 offers a summary of dosing considerations for antimicrobials in the ICU patient undergoing CRRT.

Table 20.3 provides dosing recommendations for some common antimicrobial agents used in the ICU that require dose adjustment in CRRT. Dosing recommendations are based on available literature and expert opinion, and include dose ranges to account for patient factors including body weight and severity of infection. The information in Table 20.3 includes general recommendations only and they should not supersede clinical judgment. Of note, loading doses for these drugs are not affected by the presence of CRRT because their determinant is Vd. Loading doses should be strongly considered to achieve rapid therapeutic levels.

Summary of Drug Dosing in CRRT

Drug dosing during CRRT is complicated. The important variables for consideration were discussed in this chapter. Drug clearance is highly dependent on the method of renal replacement, filter type, and flow rate. Appropriate dosing requires close monitoring of pharmacological response, signs of adverse reactions resulting from drug accumulation, as well as drug levels in relation to target peak or trough (if appropriate). When available, therapeutic drug monitoring should be applied to optimize drug therapy and limit adverse effects. The use of alternative agents that are not dependent on renal clearance or not associated with drug-induced AKI should be considered when applicable. Ensuring optimal drug efficacy and avoidance of adverse drug events requires a frequent and skillful assessment.

Key Reference

Choi G, Gomersall CD, Tian Q, Joynt GM, Freebairn RC, Lipman J. Principles of antibacterial dosing in continuous renal replacement therapy. *Crit Care Med.* 2009;37:2268–2282.

Heintz BH, Matzke GR, Dager WE. Antimicrobial dosing concepts and recommendations for critically ill adult patients receiving continuous renal replacement therapy or intermittent hemodialysis. *Pharmacotherapy.* 2009;29:562–577.

Roberts JA, Paul SK, Akova M, et al. DALI: defining antibiotic levels in intensive care unit patients: are current β-lactam antibiotic doses sufficient for critically ill patients? *Clin Infect Dis.* 2014;58:1072–1083.

Part 3

Special Situations

Chapter 21

Renal Replacement Therapy in Children

Michael L. Moritz

There are various options for renal replacement therapy (RRT) in children. The type of RRT depends largely on the child's size, the reason for initiating therapy, and the equipment and expertise available at an institution. Acute RRT is not nearly as often performed in children as it is in adults, and not all RRTs are available at each pediatric center. Peritoneal dialysis (PD) is the most widely available RRT, performed at almost all pediatrics centers. Intermittent hemodialysis (HD) is also widely available, but many centers do not have the expertise or equipment to dialyze infants or neonates. Continuous venovenous hemofiltration (CVVH) is becoming more available at pediatric centers, but is offered primarily at large pediatric tertiary care centers. RRT in the large child or adolescent (>50 kg) is no different than in adults. The focus of this chapter is to discuss RRT as it pertains to infants and small children. A complete discussion of RRTs can be found elsewhere in this manual.

Indications

The most common reasons for initiating acute RRT in children are similar to adults: fluid overload, acute kidney injury, sepsis, multisystem organ failure, solid organ transplants, and bone marrow transplants. There are some reasons for initiating RRT in children that are different than adults, such as postoperative congenital heart disease repair, urea cycle disorders, and hemolytic uremic syndrome.

Peritoneal Dialysis

PD remains an attractive form of RRT for a variety of reasons. PD catheters are relatively easy to insert and can be placed in virtually any size child. It is an inexpensive therapy that does not require sophisticated dialysis equipment or highly trained personnel. Acute PD is performed primarily after postoperative complex congenital heart disease repair. PD is a better option than CVVH in these children because of their small size and because PD does not require vascular access or systemic anticoagulation. Many cardiac centers place a PD

Box 21.1 Contraindication to Peritoneal Dialysis

- Recent abdominal surgery (5–7 days)
- Abdominal drains
- Abdominal wall defects
- Communication between abdomen and thorax
- Extensive abdominal adhesion
- Peritoneal membrane failure
- Ventriculoperitoneal shunt

NxStage continuous renal replacement therapy with hemofilter systems with low volume cartridge

System	Material	Surface area (m²)	Blood volume (mL)
HF-400	Polyarylethysulfone	0.3	83
HF-700	Polyarylethysulfone	0.71	108
HF-1200	Polyarylethysulfone	1.25	138

catheter at the time of cardiac repair and initiate PD if there is oliguria, fluid overload, or metabolic derangements.

Contraindications to PD

There are only a few contraindications to PD (Box 21.1). A gastrostomy tube, ileostomy, colostomy, and vesicostomy are not contraindications to PD. A ventriculoperitoneal shunt is a relative contraindication to PD, but should be initiated only by experienced dialysis personnel.

PD Access

A single-cuff acute Tenckoff catheter is the most common catheter used for acute PD in children. The catheters can be either straight or coiled, and they come in three sizes: infant, pediatric, and adult (Box 21.2). Pediatric and adult catheters have the same internal diameter, but only differ in length.

Apparatus for PD

Acute PD is easy to initiate. Manual PD can be initiated with a "Y-set" that connects to the PD catheter. One end of the Y is connected to the dialysate solution and the other end is connected to a drain bag. Manual PD can then be initiated. A burretrol is required to deliver small dwell volumes in infants.

Box 21.2 Selection of Acute Tenckoff Peritoneal Dialysis Catheter

- Less than 3 kg, infant catheter
- More than 3 kg and less than 20 kg, pediatric catheter
- More than or equal to 20 kg, adult catheter

> **Box 21.3 Initial Peritoneal Dialysis Prescription**
>
> • 1.5% Dextrose + 200 U heparin/L
> • 10 mL/kg dwell volume
> • Continuous hourly exchanges

A specially manufactured manual dialysis set called Daily-Nate is available for performing manual PD in small infants. Dialy-Nate is a closed system with a graded burretrol to deliver small volumes, a drain bag, multiple connectors for dialysate, and an optional heating coil. An automated cycler can be used in the larger infant. The minimum volume that can be delivered by a cycler is 60 mL. It is best to use a cycler when a dwell volume of 100 mL or greater is used.

Acute PD Prescription

There are various components to writing an acute PD prescription. Box 21.3 describes a typical prescription to initiate PD. The following sections explain each component of the dialysis prescription.

Dialysate

The dialysate solution is referred to by the dextrose concentration as either 1.5%, 2.5%, or 4.25%. Dialysate is hyperosmolar in relationship to the plasma. Uremic toxins, electrolytes and water are removed from the patient via diffusion into the peritoneum. Below are general principles for writing acute peritoneal dialysis orders at the initiation of peritoneal dialysis and the adjutments for continued peritoneal dialysis as it pertains to selecting the dialysate solution, dwell volume and dwell time.

Dialysate solution
• A 1.5% dialysate solution is the standard concentration for initiating PD.
• The dextrose concentration can be increased if additional fluid removal is required.
• A total of 200 to 500 U heparin/L are usually added to the dialysate to prevent fibrin clots.
• Heparin does not cross the peritoneum.
• A total of 2 to4 mEq/L potassium can be added to the dialysate if hypokalemia develops.

Dwell Volume

Acute PD is initiated at a low dwell volume to prevent leakage of dialysate around the catheter from higher intraperitoneal volume. The dwell volume can be increased progressively over time to improve clearance.

• PD is initiated at a dwell volume of 10 mL/kg.
• The dwell volume can be increased progressively over 2 weeks to up to 40 mL/kg.

Dwell Time
- Acute PD is usually initiated with hourly exchanges.
- Twenty- to 30-minute exchanges can be use if
  - PD is initiated within 24 hours of catheter placement
  - Aggressive fluid removal is needed
  - There is severe hyperkalemia
- Acute PD is usually continuous.
- Intermittent PD of 8 to 10 hours can be done when dwell volumes greater than 30 mL/kg are achieved.

Complications

There are a variety of complications associated with PD. The following lists the key aspects to a variety of complications:

- Leakage of fluid around the PD catheter
  - Interrupt PD for 24 to 48 hours
  - Resume at a reduced dwell volume
  - Consider administering fibrin glue to the exit site
- Peritonitis
  - Evidenced by cloudy fluid, abdominal pain, and fever.
  - Send peritoneal fluid for cell count, gram stain and culture.
  - Evidence of peritonitis on peritoneal cell count.
    - >100 WBC μL
    - >50% neutrophils
  - Treat with intraperitoneal antibiotics.
  - PD does not have to be discontinued.
- Problems with filling and draining
  - Check catheter placement on abdominal radiograph.
  - Treat constipation.
  - Consider increasing dwell volume.
  - Change position of the patient.
  - Add heparin to dialysate if fibrin is present.
  - Consider using tissue plasminogen activator (TPA)in PD catheter.
  - Consider whether omentum is wrapped around the catheter and surgical intervention is needed.

Hemodialysis

Hemodialysis (HD) is a widely available RRT in most pediatric centers. It can be performed successfully in infants weighing 2 kg or more, and in even smaller neonates by very experienced personal. Infant and neonatal HD requires special equipment and modifications in the dialysis prescription because of the small blood volume of these patients. An adult dialysis prescription with adult lines and dialyzers are not appropriate for children who

Table 21.1 Vascular access in children

Patient Size (kg)	Catheter Size
Neonate, <3	3.5-Fr or 5-Fr umbilical artery catheter
	5-Fr umbilical venous catheter
	5-Fr single-lumen venous catheters
	Radial arterial line
	7-Fr double-lumen dialysis catheter
3–6	7-Fr double-lumen dialysis catheter
6–30	8- or 9-Fr double-lumen dialysis catheter
>30	10-, 11-, or 11.5-Fr double-lumen dialysis catheter

weigh less than 40 kg. Below are general prinicples for initiating acute hemodialysis in infants and children as it relates to the selecting the appropriate vascular access, dialysis blood lines and dialyzers, blood flow rate, time of dialysis, ultrafiltration and anticoagulation.

Acute HD Access

Reliable vascular access is critical for doing HD or CVVH in children. There are a variety of HD catheter sizes available for children (Table 21.1). Dialysis is usually performed through a double-lumen hemodialysis catheter. In neonates, HD can be performed through umbilical lines or through a radial arterial line and a single-lumen central venous catheter.

Dialysis Blood Lines and Dialyzers

Dialysis blood lines and dialyzers come in a variety of sizes. The exact blood volume differs among manufacturers. Selecting an appropriate blood line and dialyzer is critical to dialyzing children (Table 21.2). When selecting a dialyzer and blood lines in a child the below guidelines should be kept in mind.

- The surface are of the dialyzer should be approximately the same as the body surface area of the child.

Table 21.2 Examples of appropriate dialysis prescriptions for children

Patient Size: Weight (kg), Body Surface Area (m²)	Blood Lines, Volume (mL)	Dialyzer, Volume (mL), Surface Area (m²)	Priming Volume (mL), % Blood Volume	Blood Flow Rate (mL)
4.0, 0.3	Neonatal, 20	F3*, 28, 0.4	48, 15	12–40
10.0, 0.5	Small pediatric, 44	F3, 28, 0.4	48, 6	30–100
30.0, 1.0	Large pediatric, 79	F5, 63, 1.0	142, 6	100–300

*F3 and F5 are manufactured by Fresenius.

- The extracorporeal volume (ECV) of the blood line and dialyzer should not exceed 10% of the patient's blood volume (8 mL/kg).
- If the ECV exceeds 10% of the blood volume, prime the lines with 5% albumin or whole blood (hematocrit, 30%–35%).

Blood Flow rate

- The first dialysis treatment should be 3 to 5 mL/kg/h.
- Subsequent dialysis treatments can be as much as 10 mL/kg/h.

Time of dialysis

- Dialysis is extremely efficient in small children because of the small volume of distribution.
- A 3-hour dialysis treatment is usually sufficient for children who weigh less than 50 kg.

Ultrafiltration rate

- Ultrafiltration should not exceed 5% to 7% of body weight in a 3-hour treatment.

Anticoagulation

- Administer a loading dose of 30 to 50 U/kg.
- Administer a continuous heparin infustion of10 U/kg hourl
- Heparin-free dialysis can be done with high blood flows and saline flushes.
- Lock catheters with 1:1000 U heparin/L.

Sustained Low-Efficiency Dialysis

Sustained low-efficiency dialysis (SLED) is beginning to emerge as a viable option for RRT in critically ill children, and some pediatric centers are adopting it. SLED is a "hybrid therapy" in which conventional HD machines and equipment are used for extended daily dialysis that lasts 6 to 18 hours. Solute and fluid removal is greater than intermittent HD and it allows for scheduled downtime. One of the major advantages of using SLED is that it requires the same equipment and dialysis staff as that used for children undergoing conventional intermittent HD. Therefore, specialized equipment, staff, and protocols for preventing bradykinin release associated with AN69 membranes are avoided. The Fresenius 2008K has a continuous renal replacement therapy (CRRT) mode with a dialysate flow of 100 mL/h, which is suitable for SLED in infants. The primary disadvantages of doing SLED in small children is that ultrafiltration is not as accurate as with CRRT machines, a dialysate flow of 100 mL/h may be excessive in an infant, and the dialysate could, in theory, expose the patient to endotoxins. As newer dialysis systems are developed, SLED may play a greater role in children in the future.

Table 21.3 Prismaflex continuous renal replacement therapy hemofilter systems

System	Material	Surface area (m²)	Blood volume (mL)
M60	Acrylonitrile	0.6	93
M100	Acrylonitrile	0.9	152
M150	Acrylonitrile	1.5	189
HF1000	Polyarylethysulfone	1.1	165
HF 1400	Polyarylethysulfone	1.4	186

Continuous Venovenous Hemofiltration

The principles of CVVH are the same for children as adults. CVVH is technically more difficult in small children than HD because of the larger priming volume of the system (Table 21.3). Ther are different systems available for doing CRRT in children and different centers will need to consider the pros and cons of each manufacturer system when deciding which system employ and physicians will need to familiarize themselves with each system in order to develop appropriate protocols. The NxStage system has the smallest system priming volume of 83 mL and uses exclusively polysufone hemofilters. The minimum priming volume for the Prismaflex system M60 set manufactured by Gambro is 93 mL. According to the manufacturer, the minimum patient weight for CVVH is 11 kg. CVVH should not be attempted in children who weigh less than 10 kg unless the center has significant experience with children of this size and an established protocol to address the large PV. The Prismaflex system uses an acrylonitrile (AN69) membrane, which have been associated with a bradykinin release syndrome when exposed to an acidic environments. Therefore, an acidic blood prime coming in contact with AN69 membranes could result in bradykinin release syndrome. This syndrome could prove fatal in critically ill infants. CVVH treatment must be stopped immediately and the system discarded without returning the blood to the patient. Therefore, a standard blood prime with packed red blood cells (PRBC), as is done for HD, should not be attempted with AN69 Prismaflex systems. The NxStage system has the advantage of only using HF filters which are not associated with bradykinin release syndrome. Different pediatric centers have proposed ways of dealing with this problem, such as the following:

• Maintaining zero-balance ultrafiltration (dialyzing the blood prime before administering it to the patient)
• Using an adult-size filter that is not AN69, such as the Prismaflex HF system, which has a polyarylethersulfone membrane with a minimum PV of 165 mL, or using the NxStage system.

- Buffering the blood prime by adding sodium bicarbonate and/or tris-hydroxymethyl aminomethane to it as it is being infused into the patient
- Doing an effective blood prime by priming the system with Plasmalyte and transfusing 50 mL PRBC as the patient is going on to the system

General Principles When Initiating CVVH

Blood Pressure

The initiation of CVVH should be delayed if there is severe hypotension and hemodynamic instability. CVVH can usually be initiated successfully if the mean arterial pressure is more than 50 mmHg.

Vascular Access

At least a 7-Fr double-lumen HD catheter should be used for CVVH in children because the minimum blood flow for most CVVH machines is 30 mL/h. Note that 7-Fr catheters are prone to kinking and may need to be replaced often (Table 21.2).

Extracorporeal Volume

The PV for the CVVH system usually exceeds 10% of the blood volume in children who weigh less than 10 kg.

- Calculate the ECV of the CVVH circuit.
- The child's hematocrit should be 30% or more before initiating CVVH.
- If the PV exceeds 8 mL/kg, some form of blood prime may be required.

Blood Flow

- Blood flows on CRRT are different than on hemodialysis. In hemodialysis the dialysate flow far exceeds the blood flow, therefor clearance is limited by the blood flow and higher blood flows resuls in higher clearance. In CRRT the blood flow usually far exceeds dialysate clearance and therefor clearance is primarily reflected by the dialysate clearance. A blood flow of 3 – 5 mL/kg/hr is appropriate for performing CRRT in childrens. Higher blood flow rates can decrease that chance of system clotting but also can results system pressures when using small cartriges. Higher blood flows also result in increased citrate exposure when using citrate for anticoagulation and increase the risk fo alkalosis and citrate lock.

Dialysate Replacement Fluid Flow Rate

The choice of using CVVH or continuous venovenous hemodialysis is center specific and there is no clear advantage of one over the other in pediatrics. There are no specific CVVH solutions for children; Accusol, Prismasate, Normocarb, Nxstage, or pharmacy-made solutions have all been used successfully. Dialysis flow in children has been adapted from what has been used in adults and adjusted to body surface area. The most widely accepted dialysate rate is 2L/1.73 m²/h. In our opinion, excellent clearance and metabolic control can be obtained with flow rates much lower than this; these large flow rates can result in alkalosis, hypokalemia, and hypophosphatemia, and may not be needed in all circumstances.

Anticoagulation

Both heparin and citrate anticoagulation have been used successfully in children, and the principles are the same as in adults. Heparin anticoagulation typically requires a 30- to 50-U/kg loading dose followed by a 10- to 20-U/kg/h maintenance dose to keep to an activated clotting time of 180 to 240 seconds or a PTT of 60 to 80 seconds. Heparin anticoagulation should be avoided if the patient is immediately postoperative, if there is active bleeding, or if the patient is anticoagulated systemically. The protocol for regional citrate anticoagulation is, for the most part, the same as for adults. The ACD-A citrate flow rate is 1.5 times the blood flow rate to keep the postfilter ionized calcium level between 0.2 mM and 0.4 mM. The calcium chloride (20 mg/mL) infusion rate is 0.1 times the ACD-A flow rate to keep systemic ionized calcium levels between 1.0 mM and 1.3 mM. The adjustments made to the ACD-A and calcium chloride flow rates to maintain the appropriate ionized calcium will be 50% less for children who weigh less than 20 kg. Citrate anticoagulation can be complicated by hypernatremia, alkalosis, and citrate lock.

Recent Innovations in Pediatric CRRT

HD and CRRT in neonates and small infants provide a particular challenge. To this end, specialized equipment and machinery are becoming available to address this unique population. A recent addition to the therapies available for Prismaflex CRRT is the HF20 membrane by Gambro. This polyarylethersulfone membrane has a circuit volume of 60 mL and a surface area of 0.2 m². The HF20 membrane is not currently available in the United States, but reports outside of the United States suggest that it can be used safely and effectively in infants and small children, usually without the need for a blood prime. Two new devices have been developed to address CRRT and HD specifically in neonates and infants. The Cardio-Renal Pediatric Dialysis Emergency Machine (or CARPEDIEM) is a new CRRT machine developed specifically to treat neonates and infants who weigh 2 to 10 kg. The CARPEDIEM has a PV of only 30 mL, miniaturized roller pumps, and an accurate ultrafiltration control via calibrated scales, with a precision of 1 g. The Newcastle Infant Dialysis and Ultrafiltration System (or NIDUS) is a dialysis machine developed specifically for infants weighing 1 to 8 kg. It has a PV of only 13 mL and uses a high-flux polysulfone membrane of 0.045 m². It is capable of dialyzing from a single lumen of a central venous line delivering a blood flow of 20 mL/min, with an adjustable ultrafiltration rate of between 0 mL/h and 60 mL/h that adjusts to microliter increments. Although these two devices are not commercially available, they are published data of successful use in infants. A device that is commercially available in the US to do ultrafiltration is the the Aquadex TM by Gambro. It has a priming volume of 30 mL and can be employed through a peripheral line. Pediatric data is emerging supporting it's use for fluid removal (Aquapheresis).

Key Reference

Ronco C, Garzotto F, Brendolan A, et al. Continuous renal replacement therapy in neonates and small infants: development and first-in-human use of a miniaturised machine (CARPEDIEM). *Lancet.* 2014;383:1807–1813.

Brophy PD, Mottes TA, Kudelka TL, et al. AN-69 membrane reactions are pH-dependent and preventable. *American journal of kidney diseases : the official journal of the National Kidney Foundation.* Jul 2001;38(1):173–178.

Bunchman TE, Maxvold NJ, Brophy PD. Pediatric convective hemofiltration: Normocarb replacement fluid and citrate anticoagulation. *American journal of kidney diseases : the official journal of the National Kidney Foundation.* Dec 2003;42(6):1248–1252.

Hackbarth RM, Eding D, Gianoli Smith C, Koch A, Sanfilippo DJ, Bunchman TE. Zero balance ultrafiltration (Z-BUF) in blood-primed CRRT circuits achieves electrolyte and acid-base homeostasis prior to patient connection. *Pediatric nephrology.* Sep 2005;20(9):1328–1333.

Kaddourah A, Goldstein SL. Renal replacement therapy in neonates. *Clinics in perinatology.* Sep 2014;41(3):517–527.

Kaur A, Davenport A. Hemodialysis for infants, children, and adolescents. *Hemodialysis international. International Symposium on Home Hemodialysis.* Jul 2014;18(3):573–582.

Sutherland SM, Alexander SR. Continuous renal replacement therapy in children. *Pediatric Nephrology.* Nov 2012;27(11):2007–2016.

Sasser WC, Dabal RJ, Askenazi DJ, et al. Prophylactic peritoneal dialysis following cardiopulmonary bypass in children is associated with decreased inflammation and improved clinical outcomes. *Congenital Heart Disease.* Mar–Apr 2014;9(2):106–115.

Chapter 22

Therapeutic Plasma Exchange in Critical Care Medicine

Joseph E. Kiss

Principles

Therapeutic plasma exchange (TPE) is the automated removal of a patient's plasma and replacement (exchange) with a suitable alternative fluid such as a solution containing albumin or fresh frozen plasma. Its intended use is for depletion of pathogenic large-molecular weight substances (>30,000–50,000 Da) present in blood plasma and/or replacement of depleted normal/beneficial substances. Smaller molecular weight compounds are not removed efficiently by TPE, but may be removed effectively by alternative extracorporeal techniques such as hemofiltration (<20,000–30,000 Da) or dialysis (<500–600 Da).

The Decision to Use TPE

The rational use of TPE is based on the following considerations:

- What is the pathophysiological role of the target macromolecule in the clinical disorder? Is there evidence of acute toxicity caused by the substance? Is the patient resistant to the usual medical and/or pharmacological therapy or does the clinical urgency demand more immediate action?
- Can the substance be removed efficiently by TPE? In general, this applies to large molecules with relatively long half-lives (reduced synthetic rate).
- Is there evidence that a reduction in levels of the offending substance is associated with improved clinical outcomes?

Clinical consultation with the appropriate provider of TPE services is recommended to address these issues and to provide management guidance, as outlined in Table 22.1.

Note, the American Society for Apheresis has published comprehensive evidence-based indications on the use of TPE in specific disease categories. The classification system and examples of substances removed are shown in Box 22.1 and Table 22.2.

Table 22.1 Decision making in therapeutic plasma exchange

	Considerations
Rationale	Disease pathogenesis, published efficacy, and quality of evidence
Technical issues	Vascular access, volume of plasma to process, replacement solution
Management plan	Timing (emergent, urgent?), number and frequency of treatments
End point	Clinical and/or laboratory response

Management Guidelines for TPE

The extent of removal of a substance during TPE depends on the volume of the patient's plasma removed in relation to total plasma volume (PV), the distribution of the substance between the intravascular and extravascular compartments, and how rapidly the substance reequilibrates between compartments. PV is calculated as PV = Total blood volume x (1 − Hematocrit level). In adults, the total blood volume may be estimated as 70mL/kg. Therefore, for a 70-kg man with a hematocrit level of 0.45 (45%), PV = 4900 mL x 0.55, or 2695 mL.

A one-compartment model best describes the kinetics of removal in TPE. The rate of removal is not linear but curvilinear (i.e., very steep during the more efficient early portion of the exchange, then leveling off during the latter portion of the procedure as more of the replacement fluid and less of the original patient's plasma is exchanged). During a TPE procedure, removal of immunoglobulin (Ig) M and fibrinogen, which are located predominantly in the intravascular compartment (~80%), is more complete than removal of IgG because only ~40% of this protein is intravascular. From a practical standpoint, IgM-mediated disorders require fewer TPE treatments to achieve a similar level of removal than IgG-mediated disorders. Lower molecular weight compounds that are highly diffusible (i.e., have a large volume of distribution) or are regulated actively in the plasma (such as calcium or potassium) are removed much less efficiently by TPE. After being depleted by TPE, the return of a substance toward baseline levels is governed by a balance of synthesis,

Box 22.1 Consensus Indications for Plasma Exchange

ASFA Category	Interpretation	Remarks
I	Standard acceptable therapy	Proved in controlled trials
II	Available evidence supports efficacy	Case series; second line, adjunctive therapy
III	Available evidence suggests efficacy but is inconclusive	Anecdotal data (e.g., case reports)
IV	Ineffective in controlled trials	

ASFA, American Society for Apheresis.

Table 22.2 Clinical examples when plasma exchange is used

Substance Removal/ Replenishment	Clinical Examples	ASFA Category
Substances removed		
Autoantibodies	Goodpasture's syndrome (antiglomerular basement membrane autoantibodies)	I
Alloantibodies	Renal transplant rejection (donor-specific anti-HLA)	I
Immunoglobulins causing hyperviscosity	Waldenstrom's macroglobulinemia	I
Cryoglobulins	Cryoglobulin-associated skin ulceration, renal dysfunction	I
Protein-bound toxins	Amanita (mushroom) poisoning	II
Substances Replenished		
ADAMTS13 (von-Willebrand factor cleaving protease)	Thrombotic thrombocytopenic purpura	I
Coagulation factors	Hepatic failure	III

ADAMTS13, a disintegrin and metalloprotease with thrombospondin type 1 motifs 13; ASFA, American Society for Apheresis; HLA, Human Leukocyte Antigen; For a comprehensive list of indications please see the ASFA guidelines.

catabolism, and reequilibration between compartments. Variability in these factors, as well as the binding characteristics of the substance, relates to the overall efficacy of a course of treatment. Box 22.2 depicts the proportion of an idealized compound that is removed based on the kinetic model.

Apheresis Devices

Two general types of instrumentation may be used to perform TPE: centrifugal-based and membrane filtration.

Box 22.2 Removal of a Substance by Therapeutic Plasma Exchange

- Efficiency
  - 1 PV = 65% removal
  - 1.5 PV = 75% removal
  - 2 PV = 87% removal
  - 3 PV = 95% removal
- IgM: 80% intravascular (efficiently depleted as a result of limited reequilibration)
- IgG: both intravascular (40%) and in tissues (removal less efficient, redistribution into plasma postapheresis over a 24- to 48-hour period)

Note: Ig, immunoglobulin; PV, plasma volume. The volume processed during therapeutic plasma exchange procedures is often "capped" at 1.5 PV because of the minimal additional effect of increasing the procedure time above this level (i. e., only 12% additional removal/replacement occurs from 1.5 to 2.0 PV).

Centrifugal Cell Separators

Centrifugal separation relies on the application of gravitational force to separate blood elements according to density. In order from lightest to heaviest, whole-blood components may be separated into plasma (Specific Gravity, 1.025–1.029), platelets (SG, 1.040), lymphocytes (SG, 1.070), granulocytes (SG, 1.087–1.092), and red blood cells (SG, 1.093–1.096). Centrifugal cell separators operate either by discontinuous flow (alternates blood collection and reinfusion sequentially) or continuous flow. Continuous flow devices achieve greater efficiency by collecting and reinfusing processed blood components simultaneously.

In a typical TPE channel configuration, whole blood is withdrawn from the patient by means of an inlet pump. To prevent clotting, it is mixed immediately with an anticoagulant solution at a preset ratio, typically 10 to 14 parts whole blood to 1 part of Acid Citrate Dextrose-A(ACD-A). The blood then enters the separation chamber, where an interface is established to separate the blood into component layers. The heavier cellular elements settle to the outside of the channel, whereas the lighter plasma remains in the inner aspect. The plasma is siphoned off through the plasma-out tube, and the cellular components are removed through the red blood cell return tube. Typical flow rates for therapeutic plasma exchange range from 60 to 95 mL/min, depending on patient size, patient tolerance of side effects, and type of replacement solution being used.

Anticoagulation

Most centrifugal cell separators use citrate anticoagulants; protocols are also available for using heparin alone or heparin and citrate in combination. Use of citrate avoids potential bleeding risks of systemic anticoagulation; however, the hypocalcemia induced by citrate has certain potentially serious toxicities, including seizures and depression of cardiac function. For this reason, manufacturers of apheresis instrumentation have designed controls that regulate the maximum amount of citrate that can be infused. The maximum AC(anticoagulant citrate) infusion rate is based on the average patient's ability to metabolize citrate under normal physiological conditions. However, many patients, such as those with liver failure, have a reduced clearance of citrate so individual factors need to be considered.

Priming of the Extracorporeal Circuit

A saline prime is used in the external tubing and channel of the apheresis instrument to avoid hypotension resulting from a sudden volume deficit. The extracorporeal volume, or "dead space volume," within the TPE circuit varies among different machines, ranging between 170 mL and 250 mL. Dilution of an adult's red blood cell mass by this volume is negligible; however, it may be substantial for a child. Red blood cell prime methods have been developed to minimize the effects of hemodilution.

Membrane Filtration Cell Separators

Membrane filtration technology is an extension of the use of synthetic biocompatible membranes used in hemodialysis, ultrafiltration, and hemofiltration. The membrane is permeable to large-molecular weight proteins but excludes cellular elements, including platelets. Pore sizes ranging from 0.2 to 0.6 μm allow passage of proteins with molecular weights of more than 500,000 Da. Membrane filters in current use have sieving coefficients of 0.9 to 1.0, meaning the protein composition of the filtrate and the plasma are nearly identical, even for very large molecules such as IgM. Cellulose diacetate, polyethylene, polypropylene, polyvinylchloride, and other synthetic materials are used.

After the addition of an anticoagulant, the patient's blood is pumped through either a parallel plate or a hollow fiber filter at a continuous flow rate between 50 mL/min and 200 mL/min. The efficiency of filtration is determined by several parameters, including the blood flow rate, composition and physical characteristics of the membrane, transmembrane pressure, geometry of the blood flow path, as well as the physical and chemical nature of the plasma proteins. A typical device features an anticoagulant syringe pump (usually using heparin as the anticoagulant of choice), a blood pump, replacement fluid pump, and effluent pump. Blood is directed to the plasma filter by means of the blood pump. The hemoconcentrated blood leaves the plasma filter through the return line, where it is combined with replacement fluid and returned to the patient. The effluent side of the plasma filter leads to a waste bag.

Studies comparing centrifugal and membrane filtration have found them to be similar with respect to safety and efficiency. TPE is not as rapid with membrane separators. Although use of systemic heparin anticoagulation may avoid some side effects of citrate, systemic heparinization is disadvantageous in some patients, such as those with coagulopathy.

Adverse Effects of TPE

Serious complications such as infection, thrombosis, pneumothorax, and hematoma formation are often related to the need for central venous access. Overall, 3% to 8% of TPE procedures may be associated with adverse reactions (Table 22.3). Most of these reactions are easily recognized and treated. Severe reactions, such as cardiac or respiratory arrest, and mortality (1–2/10,000 procedures) are rare. The more serious consequences are seldom a result of the TPE procedure itself. The lists that follow provide more information on the adverse effects of TPE.

Approximate Rate Based on Published Literature
• There is a higher rate associated with TPE in which plasma is used.

Table 22.3 Adverse events and frequency	
Event	Frequency* (%)
Overall rate	7.81 (with plasma replacement); 3.35 (no plasma)
Specific reaction rates	
Transfusion reactions (resulting primarily from plasma replacement)	1.6
Citrate-related nausea and/or vomiting (paresthesias higher rate)	1.2
Hypotension‡	1.0
Vasovagal nausea and/or vomiting	0.5
Pallor and/or diaphoresis	0.5
Tachycardia	0.4
Respiratory distress	0.3
Tetany or seizure	0.2

*Specific reactions rates are listed for all therapeutic apheresis procedures, however, the majority were TPE. Reference: McLeod BC, et al. Transfusion. 1999;39:282-8. ‡Systolic blood pressure < 80 mm Hg.

- Autonomic dysfunction with hypotension is seen, especially in patients treated for neurological conditions, including Guillain-Barré syndrome and chronic idiopathic demyelinating polyneuropathy

Citrate Toxicity

- One part acid citrate dextrose solution is added to 14 parts whole blood immediately after withdrawal from the patient to prevent clotting in the apheresis machine. The citrate ions bind ionized calcium, resulting in transient hypocalcemia. Plasma products add to this side effect because of high citrate concentration.

  - Symptoms
    - Perioral tingling
    - Vibration sensation
    - Numbness and tingling in extremities
    - Nausea and emesis
    - Possible progression to muscle spasms, tetany, and seizure activity
  - Management
    - Decrease inlet flow (blood withdrawal) rate (or pause machine).
    - Administer a calcium gluconate infusion. In adults, 10 mL 10% (1 g) in 250 mL Normal Salinr Solution(NSS) or may be added to albumin replacement fluid (not plasma!).
    - Administer a calcium chloride infusion. In adults, this is three times more potent and faster acting than calcium gluconate because the ions dissociate immediately. Monitor patients' [Ca^{2+}] levels every 15 to 30 minutes.
  - Vasovagal reactions

- Generally manifested by sudden hypotension and bradycardia, diaphoresis, lightheadedness, and occasionally nausea and emesis
- TPE halted temporarily and legs elevated to increase venous return
- Reaction usually self-limited but may progress to loss of consciousness
- Bolus NSS, 200 to 400 mL, may be given
- Hypotension
  - Acute volume loss is prevented by priming the apheresis circuit with replacement fluid.
  - Despite simultaneous replacement, patients such as those with autonomic neuropathy are sensitive and become hypotensive.
  - Generally responds to bolus NSS, 200 to 400 mL.
- Allergic reactions
  - Mainly resulting from plasma proteins
  - Rarely albumin or residual ethylene oxide sterilization of disposable plastic
- Hemolysis
  - Very rare
  - Suspect use of hypotonic crystalloid solution or mechanical cause (kinked tubing), or patient red blood cell abnormality
- Depletion of clotting factors
  - Prolonged PT, INR, and/or APTT that occur with daily serial TPE using nonplasma replacement or cryodepleted plasma (Table 22.4)
  - TPE depletes fibrinogen especially—longer half-life (90 hours) and slower recovery rate than other coagulation factors (3–4 days to return to normal)
- Usually not manifest with every-other-day plasma exchanges
- Treatment is to decrease frequency of procedures or use plasma or cryoprecipitate (donor exposure risk)
- Transfusion-transmitted diseases (when plasma used)—rare

Table 22.4 Colloid replacement fluids used in therapeutic plasma exchange

Fluid	Advantages	Disadvantages
5% Albumin	Viral inactivation	High cost
	Ease of use	Most proteins not replaced
	Reactions rare	
Single-donor plasma*	All proteins replaced	High cost
		Inconvenient†
		Citrate reactions
		Urticaria
		Viral infection risk

*Fresh frozen plasma or cryoprecipitate-poor plasma.

†Must be thawed before use and must match patient ABO type.

- Angiotensin-converting enzyme (ACE) inhibitors
  - Symptoms
    - Flushing (vasodilation), hypotension, dyspnea, watery diarrhea
    - Prekallikrein activator (an activator of bradykinin) present in albumin-containing replacement solutions
    - ACE identical to kinase II; bradykinin degradation inhibited
  - Prevention includes withholding ACE inhibitors at least 24 hours before a procedure.

Key References

Schwartz J, Winters JL, Padmanabhan A, et al. Guidelines on the use of therapeutic apheresis in clinical practice: evidence-based approach from the Writing Committee of the American Society for Apheresis: the sixth special issue. *J Clin Apheresis.* 2013;28(3):145–284.

Szczepiorkowski ZM. Clinical applications of therapeutic apheresis: an evidence based approach. *J Clin Apheresis.* 2007;22:96–105.

Chapter 23

MARS

Molecular Adsorbent Recirculating System

Nigel Fealy and Rinaldo Bellomo

The Molecular Adsorbent Recirculating System (MARS) is an artificial liver support system aimed at the removal of toxins in patients with acute liver failure (ALF) or acute on chronic liver failure (AoCLF). MARS is used via an additional circuit attached to a standard extracorporeal circuit (continuous renal replacement circuit), which uses albumin as a dialysis medium. Using albumin as carrier molecule, toxins are then adsorbed onto specific sorbents. Most liver toxins such as bilirubin, ammonia, fatty acids, hydrophobic bile acids, and nitric oxide use albumin as their transport protein and, as a result, appear to be removed more effectively by an albumin-enriched dialysate. This albumin dialysate is regenerated online by passage through a second hemodialyzer and two sorbent columns (charcoal and an anion exchanger).

Method

The MARS treatment kit consists of an albumin hemodialyzer, a standard hemodialyzer, an activated carbon adsorber and an anion exchanger. The circuit is filled with 500 mL 20% human albumin solution. Albumin acts as dialysate and is pumped through a hollow fiber membrane (MARS flux dialyzer) countercurrent to blood (Figure 23.1, point A). Water-soluble substances diffuse into the albumin solution while albumin-bound toxins move by physicochemical interactions among plasma, albumin molecules bound to the dialysis side of the membrane, and the circulating albumin solution.

Toxin-carrying albumin is then passed through another hemodialyzer countercurrent to a standard buffered dialysis solution where diffusive clearance of water-soluble substances occurs (Figure 23.1, point B). A concentration gradient is maintained by circulation of the albumin solution and disposal of the albumin-bound toxins by passage through activated charcoal (Figure 23.1, point C), and anion exchange columns (Figure 23.1, point D) (Figure 23.2).

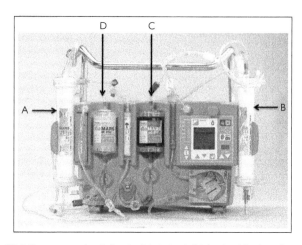

Figure 23.1 Extracorporeal and albumin dialysis circuit (Molecular Adsorbent Recirculating System [MARS]monitor). A, MARS flux dialyzer; B, standard high-flux hemodialyzer; C, activated charcoal; D, anion exchange column.

Practical Considerations

The MARS treatment is achieved by the combined use of a standalone continuous renal replacement therapy (CRRT) machine or hemodialysis machine, and the MARS albumin pump and monitor unit. The MARS albumin pump and monitor unit (Figure 23.3, point A) is placed in series with a standard

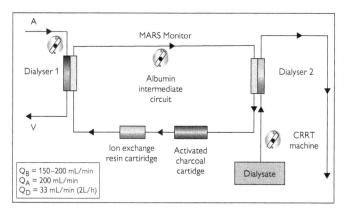

Figure 23.2 Schematic representation of a Molecular Adsorbent Recirculating System circuit. A, outflow lumen of dialysis catheter; CRRT, continuous renal replacement therapy; Q_A, albumin flow; Q_B, blood flow; Q_D, dialysate flow; V, inflow lumen of dialysis catheter.

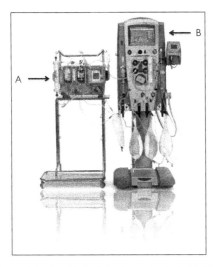

Figure 23.3 Molecular Adsorbent Recirculating System (MARS) with Prisma continuous renal replacement therapy machine. A, MARS unit; B, = Prisma continuous renal replacement therapy machine.

continuous venovenous hemodialysis circuit (Figure 23.1, point B). Depending on the external CRRT or dialysis machine used, the CRRT machine may act as a blood pump and dialysate controller or is more integrated for MARS use, as with the Prisma or Prismaflex machines (Figure 23.3, with Prisma).

As with other renal replacement therapies, suitable vascular access is a key factor in achieving the prescribed treatment dose. The use of anticoagulation should be considered carefully. Often, patients with ALF have some degree of autoanticoagulation and do not require anticoagulants to maintain MARS or CRRT circuits. And, often, the difficulty in treating patients with ALF is determining when to institute MARS therapy, duration of therapy (intermittent vs. continuous), and when to cease therapy. Box 23.1 outlines one set of recommendations for the use of MARS in ALF.

After 3 days of consecutive intermittent or continuous treatments there is an expectation that the patient with ALF or AoCLF will have significant improvement both clinically and biochemically.

Currently there are insufficient data to demonstrate a survival benefit when MARS is instituted in patients with ALF or AoCLF. However, there is evidence to suggest that MARS impacts favorably on the complications of liver failure. MARS appears to improve several clinical parameters such as hemodynamic status, bilirubin levels, bile acid levels, encephalopathy, pruritus, and renal function. The effect of improving these parameters in patients with liver failure is to provide time for either liver regeneration or to bridge the patient safely to liver transplantation.

> ### Box 23.1 Guidelines for the Use of the Molecular Adsorbent Recirculating System (MARS) in Liver Failure
>
> **Start Criteria**
>
> Increasing total bilirubin greater than 300 μmol/L *and* one of the following:
> - Hepatic encephalopathy of grade II or greater or
> - Hepatorenal syndrome
>
> **Intermittent MARS Treatment**
>
> - Six to 8 hour of treatment with intermittent hemodialysis
> - Use when hemodynamically stable and no evidence of cerebral edema
> - Anticoagulation—none, heparin, or citrate (risk of citrate accumulation)
> - Blood flow rate (Q_B) at 250 mL/min
> - Albumin flow rate (Q_A) at 250 mL/min
>
> **Continuous MARS Treatment**
>
> - Twenty-four hours of treatment with continuous venovenous hemodialysis
> - Use when hemodynamically unstable or evidence of cerebral edema
> - Anticoagulation—none, heparin, or citrate (risk of citrate accumulation)
> - Q_B at 180 to 200 mL/min
> - Q_A at 180 to 200 mL/min
>
> **Stop Criteria**
>
> Plan for at least 3 days of MARS treatment. Stop when
> - Total bilirubin less than 200 μmol/L or
> - Resolution of hepatic encephalopathy

A consideration when applying the therapy is modification of antibiotics and drug therapy. Theoretically, removal of both water-soluble and albumin-bound drugs is achieved during MARS therapy, and therefore adjustment of drug therapy and therapeutic drug level monitoring should be undertaken.

The exposure of blood to an extracorporeal circuit initiates the coagulation cascade and may deplete clotting factors and lower the platelet count. In patients with an impaired coagulation state, observation of bleeding and investigation of platelet count should be undertaken during treatments and before recommencement of MARS therapy.

Clinical application of MARSMARS continues to be the most frequently used liver support therapy in critically ill patients. It is a technically feasible therapeutic option for liver support in the intensive care environment. However, the setup is labor intensive in comparison with CRRT. This treatment option is currently limited to intensive care units in specialist referral centers where highly skilled nurses are available to institute and maintain the therapy.

MARS appears to allow for safe removal of albumin-bound and water-bound toxic substances in patients with AoCLF and ALF. Currently, many physicians believe that MARS is a useful "bridge" to transplantation or in supporting patients to recovery. As reports of clinical and biochemical improvements in patients continue to emerge, there will be continued interest in this therapy.

Key References

Boyle M, Kurtovic J, Bihari D, Riordan S, Steiner C. Equipment review: the Molecular Adsorbent Recirculating System (MARS). *Crit Care*. 2004;8(4):280–286.

Cruz D, Bellomo R, Kellum J, de Cal M, Ronco C. The future of extracorporeal support. *Crit Care Med*. 2008;36(4):s243–s252.

Evenpoel P, Laleman W, Wilmer A, et al. Prometheus versus Molecular Adsorbent Recirculating System: comparison of efficiency in two different liver detoxification devices. *Artif Organs*. 2006;30(4):276–284.

Fealy N, Baldwin I, Boyle M. The Molecular Adsorbent Recirculating System (MARS). *Austr Crit Care*. 2005;18(3):96–102.

Mitzner S. Albumin dialysis: an update. *Curr Opin Nephrol Hypertens*. 2007;16:589–595.

Nevens F, Laleman W. Artificial liver support devices as treatment option for liver failure. *Best Pract Res Clin Gastroenterol*. 2012;26:17–26.

Tsipotis E, Shuja A, Jaber BL. Albumin dialysis for liver failure: A systematic review. Advances in Chronic Kidney Disease. 2015, 22(5):382–390

Phua J, Hoe Lee K. Liver support devices. *Curr Opin Crit Care*. 2008;14:208–215.

Stadlbauer V, Jalan R. Acute liver failure: liver support therapies. *Curr Opin Crit Care*. 2007;13:215–221.

Chapter 24

Sorbents

Dehua Gong and Claudio Ronco

Introduction

The possibility of removing solutes from blood to obtain blood purification has mainly focused over the years on classic hemodialysis. However, both the characteristics of some solutes that make their removal difficult, and the limited efficiency of some dialysis membranes, have spurred a significant interest in the use of further mechanisms of solute removal such as adsorption. Materials with high capacity of adsorption (sorbents) have been utilized for about 50 years in extracorporeal blood treatments of acute poisoning or uremia. With the recognition of the role of cytokines in systemic inflammatory response syndrome(SIRS) and sepsis, and the fact that most cytokines are poorly removable by conventional diffusive or convective blood purification modalities, treatment of sepsis based on sorbent technique has recently been explored.

Target Substances for Removal by Sorbent in Sepsis

Endotoxin

Endotoxin is a lipopolysaccharide (LPS) and an outer membrane molecule essential for virtually all Gram-negative bacteria. It is generally considered a major causative agent in Gram-negative bacteria infection-related shock. LPS binds to LPS-binding protein and is transferred to bind to surface molecule CD14 when it enters into blood, presented in aggregate form or monomeric form. The signal of LPS combination with CD14 is relayed by toll-like receptors to activate nuclear factor κB and produce multiple cytokines.

Superantigen

Superantigen (SAg), which is a secreted product of Gram-positive bacteria, plays an important role in activating and regulating the innate immune system. SAg is also known to be associated with toxic shock in Gram-positive bacterial infections. Unlike conventional antigens, SAg bypasses normal antigen processing steps, binds directly as an intact protein to major histocompatability complex class II molecules on the surface of antigen-presenting cells and T-cell receptors, and activates many more T cells than conventional antigens. SAg is the most powerful T-cell mitogen ever discovered. Activated T cells then produce and release massive levels of proinflammatory cytokines.

Cytokines

Activation of the immune system is almost present in all critically ill patients, particularly in patients with infection. During the early stages of immune activation, there is production and release of many proinflammatory mediators, especially tumor necrosis factor α (TNF-α), interleukin (IL) 6, IL-1, and IL-8. These cytokines augment the body's response to the pathogen and result in systemic adaptation. At the same time, an anti-inflammatory mechanism is also initiated, which includes production of IL-10, transforming growth factor β, and IL-13. If the overresponsiveness of the immune system is still uncontrolled and persists for a period, tissue damage and organ failure occur, and the anti-inflammatory effect outweighs the proinflammatory effect, leading to immunoparalysis.

Selectivity of Sorbent Used for Removal of Target Substance

According to the selectivity of target substance removal, sorbents can be divided into three groups: unselective porous particles, relative selective adsorption, and selective adsorption.

Unselective Porous Particles

This kind of sorbent consists primarily of porous polymers, such as resin, or activated charcoal. Sorbents exist in granules, spheres, cylindrical pellets, flakes, and powder. They are solid particles with a single-particle diameter between 0.05 cm and 1.2 cm. The surface area-to-volume ratio is extremely high in sorbent particles, which varies from 300 to 1200 m^2/g. They can also be defined as macroporous (pore size, >500 Å, or 50 nm), mesoporous (pore size, 20–500 Å), and microporous (pore size, <20 Å). Usually they adsorb molecules onto their surface nonspecifically by Van der Waals forces, electrostatic attraction, or hydrophobic affinity. Because molecules adsorbed onto the porous surface of a sorbent must first pass through the pores, manipulating the pore size can, to some extent, control the molecules for removal.

Relative Selective Adsorption

Recent advancements in techniques make it possible to develop many new sorbents by immobilizing a ligand specific to a certain group of substances onto matrix fibers or particles. These kinds of sorbents include Lixelle, CTR adsorber (Kaneka Corporation, Osaka, Japan), and CYT-860 (Toray Industries, Inc., Tokyo, Japan). They use hydrogen bonds or hydrophobic interactions between ligand moiety and protein chemical groups to enhance protein adsorption capacity, and use designed pore size distribution to specify the molecular weight of proteins that can be adsorbed. An SAg-adsorbing device, which is prepared from a polystyrene-based composite fiber reinforced with polypropylene, is recently undergoing investigation.

Selective Adsorption

Sorbents made by immobilization of more specific ligands onto a matrix can target the adsorption on one certain substance or limit the adsorption within a very narrow range. An adsorber composed of Polymyxin B-immobilized fibers (PMX) has been used for adsorption of endotoxins in sepsis. Adsorbers based on macroporous beads immobilized with human serum albumin such as MATISSE also aim at endotoxin adsorption. The microsphere-based detoxification system provides a platform where anti-TNF-α antibodies are immobilized onto microparticles with a diameter range of 1 to 10 μm. This system is designed to adsorb serum TNF-α during early stages of sepsis.

Efficiency of Adsorption

When a liquid mixture is brought into contact with a microporous solid, adsorption of certain components in the mixture takes place on the internal surface of the solid. The maximum extent of adsorption occurs when equilibrium is reached. No theory for predicting adsorption curves has been embraced universally. Instead, laboratory experiments must be performed at a fixed temperature (separation processes are energy intensive and affect entropy) for each liquid mixture and adsorbent to provide data for plotting curves called *adsorption isotherms* (Figure 24.1). Adsorption isotherms can be used to determine the amount of adsorbent required to remove a given amount of solute from the solvent. Another measure of the efficiency of the unit is obtained by using marker molecules to determine the so-called mass transfer zone. The mass transfer zone is the portion of the cartridge length

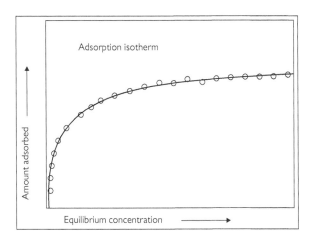

Figure 24.1 Typical example of an adsorption isotherm.

that goes from a fully saturated sorbent to a completely unsaturated condition. Mass transfer zone determination also helps to define the design of the unit and the expected time of efficiency before saturation.

Both adsorption isotherms and the mass transfer zone, however, are not a clinical practical parameter to evaluate a sorbent's adsorptive capacity. An extraction ratio is often used to reflect the removal ability of a sorbent, which is defined as the reduction ratio of solute concentration in blood or plasma after a single pass through the sorbent. Factors other than the sorbent per se also affect the extraction ratio, including blood or plasma flow rate, target solute burden in blood, and so on. In one treatment session, dynamic monitoring of the extraction ratio may reflect the saturation status of the sorbent. Another clinical useful parameter for demonstration of the removal effect of sorbents is the reduction ratio of solutes during one treatment session. However, the fact that both of these parameters cannot reflect accurately the removal ability of a sorbent makes the comparison among different sorbents difficult.

Biocompatibility of Sorbents

The concept of sorbent biocompatibility has three meanings. First, the sorbent must be resistant and release no harmful substances into body. Second, the contact of the sorbent with plasma or blood should not induce activation of complement, immune system, and hemostasis, and should not result in a hematological abnormality such as hemolysis, leukopenia, or thrombocytopenia. Third, the adsorption should not result in unwanted loss, such as albumin loss. However, so far, no one sorbent fully adheres to all these requirements.

A commercial sorbent column usually contains a sieving device that allows free passage of blood but retains particles or their fragments to prevent dissemination of small particles in the body. Some systems also include a monitoring device to detect the possible detached microparticle in the blood.

Blood–surface reaction depends on sorbent surface flatness and materials. Sometimes, a surface coating technique is used to improve sorbent biocompatibility, although at the price of adsorption efficiency. Another way to improve biocompatibility is plasma adsorption, in which only plasma passes through the sorbent, blood cells are separated from plasma and bypass the sorbent, and finally blood is reconstituted after an extracorporeal single-pass treatment. However, addition of plasma separator makes the procedure more complex. Research on materials with high molecular weight and polymers provide hope for a new type of sorbent with good biocompatibility. The new sorbent should have high selectivity of adsorption and the least unwanted loss.

Typical Modalities for the Use of Sorbents

Typical modalities for the use of sorbents in extracorporeal therapies are represented in Figure 24.2.

Hemoperfusion

Hemoperfusion is a technique in which a sorbent is placed in direct contact with blood in extracorporeal circulation. It has a very simple circuit, but requires a very biocompatible sorbent and adequate anticoagulation of the

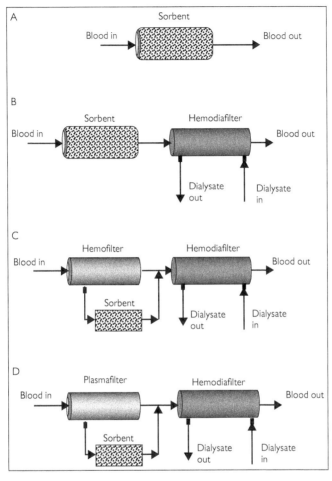

Figure 24.2 Possible modes of application of sorbents. (A) Hemoperfusion. (B) The sorbent unit is placed in series before the hemodialyzer (hemoperfusion–hemodialysis). (C) The sorbent unit is placed online in the ultrafiltrate produced from a hemofilter. The hemofilter is placed in series with the hemodialyzer. The system is used for online hemodiafiltration in chronic patients and it is defined as paired filtration dialysis with sorbent. (D) The sorbent unit is placed online in the plasma filtrate produced from a plasma filter. The plasma filter is placed in series with the hemodiafilter. The system is used for critically ill patients with septic shock and it is defined as coupled plasma filtration adsorption.

extracorporeal circuit. Materials such as charcoal, which has poor biocompatibility, must be coated before use in hemoperfusion. More recently, synthetic polymers have been introduced with a remarkable capacity for adsorption and better biocompatibility.

Hemoperfusion Coupled with Hemodialysis

Sorbents have also been used in conjunction with hemodialysis (hemoperfusion–hemodialysis). In this case, the sorbent is placed in the circuit just before the hemodialyzer, with the expectation that, after dialysis, it maintain the desired temperature or correct other abnormalities induced by the sorbent (e.g., acidosis). This modality is used mostly for removal of molecules such as beta-2 microglobulin that are poorly removed by dialysis. Another approach consists of using sorbents in "uncoated" form. These, however, cannot be placed in direct contact with whole blood and they are used for the treatment online of the ultrafiltrate or the plasma filtrate.

Double-Chamber Hemodiafiltration

In these system, plasma water is separated from whole blood and, after passing through the sorbent, it is reinfused into the blood circuit, reconstituting the whole-blood structure. This technique has been used primarily in chronic dialysis as a particular form of hemodiafiltration.

Coupled Plasma Filtration Adsorption

Continuous plasma filtration adsorption is a modality of blood purification in which plasma is separated from whole blood and circulated in a sorbent cartridge. After the sorbent unit, plasma is returned to the blood circuit and the whole blood undergoes hemofiltration or hemodialysis. The rationale consists of combining the advantages of adsorption and hemofiltration or hemodialysis techniques in solute elimination. This technique has been used mostly in septic patients showing specific advantages of blood purification, restoration of hemodynamics, and immunomodulation.

In another technique using uncoated sorbents (detoxification plasma filtration; HemoCleanse, Inc., West Lafayette, IN), a hemodiabsorption mechanism is associated with a push–pull plasma filtration system (a suspension of powdered sorbents surrounding 0.5-μm plasma filter membranes). Bidirectional plasma flow (at 80–100 mL/min) across the plasma filtration membrane provides direct contact between plasma proteins and powdered sorbents, as well as clearance of cytokines.

A major criticism may be raised concerning the removal of beneficial substances or drugs by the mechanism of adsorption. In an in vitro experiment, a hydrophobic resin sorbent was investigated for the adsorptive properties of different commonly used antibiotics. Except for vancomycin, for which a modest removal was observed, the blood levels of other antibiotics such as tobramycin or amikacin tended to remain stable over time.

Sorbents in Sepsis

Conventional blood purification has been evidenced to be less effective in removing pathogenic factors and mediators involved in the process of sepsis. This fact has aroused many innovative approaches such as high-volume hemofiltration, the use of superpermeable membranes, as well as sorbent based membranes.

Hemoperfusion using PMX is one purpose of eliminating serum endotoxins, with a reported reduction ratio of endotoxins after a single treatment of 27% to 33%.

The impact on cytokines and other mediators still remains controversial. A recent systematic review shows that hemoperfusion with PMX appears to have favorable effects on MAP, dopamine use, PaO_2/FiO_2 ratios, and mortality. Evidence from Japanese researchers suggests a blood flow rate of 80–100 mL/min and a duration of 2 hours. Possible indication requires patients to fulfill all of the following three conditions:

1. Endotoxemia or suspected Gram-negative infection
2. systemic infl ammatory response syndrome (SIRS)
3. Septic shock that necessitates vasopressor therapy

Other endotoxin adsorbers such as albumin-based sorbents have shown a trend in improvement of clinical outcome, and we await future clinical trial results.

Continuous plasma filtration adsorption is aimed at nonselective removal of soluble mediators involved in septic shock. A limited number of clinical studies have shown a beneficial effect on hemodynamics and monocyte function.

Novel sorbents are being developed for enhanced, more selective removal of cytokines, including Lixelle, CTR adsorber, CYT-860. Animal experiments have shown ability of cytokines removal, and improvement of animal survival in sepsis models. Adsorbers targeting specific removal of SAg's and TNF-α are also limited in animal experiments. These novel sorbents may soon be clinically available.

Key References

Bellomo R, Tetta C, Ronco C. Coupled plasma filtration adsorption. *Intensive Care Med.* 2003;29(8):1222–1228.

Cohen J. The immunopathogenesis of sepsis. *Nature.* 2002;420:885–891.

Cruz DN, Perazella MA, Bellomo R, et al. Effectiveness of Polymyxin B-immobilized fiber column in sepsis: a systematic review. *Crit Care.* 2007;11(2):R47.

Poll T, Opal SM. Host–pathogen interactions in sepsis. *Lancet Infect Dis.* 2008;8:32–43.

Ronco C, Brendolan A, Dan M, et al. Adsorption in sepsis. *Kidney Int Suppl.* 2000;76:S148–S155.

Ronco C, Brendolan A, d'Intini V, et al. Coupled plasma filtration adsorption: rationale, technical development and early clinical experience. *Blood Purif.* 2003;21(6):409–416.

Ronco C, Tetta C. Extracorporeal blood purification: more than diffusion and convection. Does this help? *Curr Opin Crit Care.* 2007;13:662–667.

Sakata H, Yonekawa M, Kawamura A. Blood purification therapy for sepsis. *Transfus Apher Sci.* 2006;35(3):245–251.

Shimizu T, Endo Y, Tsuchihashi H, et al. Endotoxin apheresis for sepsis. *Transfus Apher Sci.* 2006;35:271–282.

Sriskandan S, Altmann DM. The immunology of sepsis. *J Pathol.* 2008;214:211–223.

Tsuchida K, Yoshimura R, Nakatani T, et al. Blood purification for critical illness: cytokines adsorption therapy. *Ther Apher Dial.* 2006;10(1):25–31.

Chapter 25

Hybrid Therapies

Claudio Ronco, Silvia De Rosa, and Sara Samoni

General Features of Hybrid Therapies

The "hybrid therapy" is a bridge between continuous and intermittent renal replacement therapy (RRT) combining therapeutic advantages of one with cost advantages of other. General features of hybrid therapies include (1) use of standard equipment from end-stage renal disease programs, including machinery, filters, extracorporeal blood circuitry, and online fluid production for dialysate and ultrafiltrate replacement; (2) intentionally "discontinuous" therapy (i.e., intended duration is less than 24 hours); and (3) a treatment duration longer than conventional intermittent hemodialysis (IHD). Solute and fluid removal are slower than conventional IHD, but faster than conventional continuous renal replacement therapy (CRRT), thereby allowing scheduled downtime without compromise of total daily dialysis dose. Solute removal is largely diffusive, but variants with a convective component, such as sustained low-efficiency daily diafiltration (SLEDD-f) and accelerated veno-venous hemofiltration (AVVH), are possible.

Brief Orders

Session length: Six to 18 hours

Blood flow: A total of 70 to 350 mL/min

Filter: Synthetic biocompatible membrane, either low or high flux

Dialysis solution composition: For sessions lasting less than 8 hours, use sodium, 135 to 145 mEq/L; potassium, 2 to 3 mEq/L; bicarbonate, 28 to 32 mEq/L; and calcium, 1.5 to 2.5 mmol/L. For sessions lasting 8 hours or longer, use sodium, 135 to 145 mEq/L; potassium, 4 mEq/L; bicarbonate, 24 to 28 mEq/L; and calcium, 1.5 to 2.5 mmol/L

Phosphate: See text

Dialysis solution flow rate: 70–300 mL/min

Substitution fluid flow rate (for SLEDDf): 100 mL/min (with a dialysate flow (Q_D) of 200 mL/min)

Fluid removal: Determined by clinical need

Anticoagulation orders: A total of 1000 to 2000 U unfractionated heparin as bolus, then continuous infusion of 500–1000 U/h to keep activated partial thromboplastine time (aPTT) 1.5 times control

Regional citrate anticoagulation: Many protocols exist
Timing of treatment: Diurnal or nocturnal

Details of Prescription

Session Length

A number of factors help determine the prescribed duration of RRT session, such as the tolerance to ultrafiltration. Patients who are less hemodynamically stable fare better with slower ultrafiltration rates and longer treatments. Machine-related issues may also play a role, in conjunction with dialysate flow rates. For instance, for most single-pass hemodialysis machines, a single canister of dialysate concentrate lasts approximately 5 to 6 hours with a dialysate flow of 300 mL/min, or 16 to 17 hours at a dialysate flow of 100 mL/min. When the Fresenius 2008H is not equipped with CRRT software, the session length cannot be set beyond 8 hours and gives frequent alarms when treatment duration exceeds the set time. In the case of a batch system, such as the Fresenius Genius machine, a 75-L tank of dialysate lasts approximately 18 hours with a dialysate flow of 70 mL/min, and a 90-L tank lasts about 8 to 12 hours at dialysate flows of 150 to 200 mL/min.

Blood Flow

Blood flows used in the literature generally range from 70 to 350 mL/min. Interestingly, in a retrospective analysis of 100 hemodynamically unstable critically ill patients with either acute kidney injury or ESRD who received AVVH, emerged that the blood flow rate was set at 400 mL/min, as vascular access permitted. Among these patients, 79% were on vasopressors and only 5% of treatments were terminated early as a result of patient instability. Although it is common practice to prescribe a lower blood flow in ICU patients to improve cardiovascular stability, presumably by decreasing clearance and associated solute and fluid shifts, this may be less relevant during hybrid therapy. When dialysate flow is significantly lower than blood flow, as is often the case during hybrid therapy, dialysate is saturated with solute. Therefore, lowering the blood flow does not reduce solute and fluid shifts materially. On the other hand, the downside of a low blood flow is a propensity for clotting in the extracorporeal circuit. Some experts recommend maximizing blood flow as tolerated by the catheter to improve circuit patency.

Dialysis Solution Composition

As with all RRT in the ICU, the dialysate solution composition should be customized to patient needs. With prolonged treatments, a lower bicarbonate level may be preferable to avoid inducing alkalosis. In acidotic patients, a more "standard" bicarbonate bath of 35 mEq/L may be used initially, and adjusted subsequently after the initial acidosis has been corrected.

Hypophosphatemia may occur during hybrid therapy, particularly when performed daily, and phosphate levels should be monitored. To avoid this problem, one may add phosphate to the dialysate by adding 45 mL Fleet Phosphosoda to 9.5 L of bicarbonate bath (final concentration, 0.8 mmol/L) after the first few days of therapy. Alternatively, instead of manipulating the dialysate concentration, one may give phosphate supplementation, approximately 0.1 to 0.2 mmol/kg/day.

For online production of dialysate, special attention to water treatment is recommended. This is discussed later in the chapter.

Dialysis Solution Flow Rate (Variable)

In literature, dialysate flow rates r range from 70 to 300 mL/min. In general, the shorter the duration of RRT—for instance, 6 to 10 hours—the higher the dialysate flow rate (e.g., 300 mL/min) and vice versa. It is also determined in part by individual machine capabilities. Most machines frequently used for hybrid therapies do not require any adjustment for a dialysate flow of 300 mL/min or more. Minor changes in settings while in service mode can be done with the Fresenius 2008H, whereas some improvisation is necessary for the 4008H and the Gambro 200S Ultra (Table 25.1). In the case of the Fresenius Genius system, a single roller pump with two pump segments circulate blood and dialysate in either a 1:1 or 1:2 ratio.

Fluid Removal

Net ultrafiltration rate is determined by patient need and hemodynamic stability. When the Fresenius 2008H is not provided with specific CRRT software, there is a mandatory lower limit of 70 mL/h, below which frequent low-transmembrane pressure alarms may occur.

Anticoagulation Orders

Unfractionated heparin is the most commonly used anticoagulant in regimens similar to those used for conventional IHD. Heparin-free treatments are possible with the use of periodic saline flushes, but such treatments are, nevertheless, complicated by clotting of the extracorporeal circuit in a substantial proportion of cases. Clinical evidence suggests that the incidence of clotting may be slightly less with the Fresenius Genius machine, possibly related to the absence of the air-trap chamber. In hybrid therapies using convection, such as SLEDD-f and AVVH, infusion of replacement fluid in predilution mode helps abrogate hemofilter clotting but also decreases effective clearance.

There have been several descriptions of successful use of regional citrate anticoagulation for hybrid therapies for both single-pass and batch machines. Two regimens involve the use of custom calcium-free dialysate in conjunction with 4% sodium citrate solution in the arterial line. Calcium chloride is infused into the venous line.

An alternative for patients with heparin-induced thrombocytopenia is the direct thrombin inhibitor argatroban. In the absence of liver failure, a bolus of 250 μg is given, followed by an infusion of 2 μg/kg during the treatment.

Table 25.1 Hybrid therapy using various hemodialysis machines

Machine	Q_D (mL/min)	Comments
Fresenius 2008H	≥300	No adjustment needed
	100	Activate "slow dialysis" option while in service mode
		To avoid persistent low dialysate temperature alarms, recalibrate temperature control to 37°C while in service mode
		To optimize conductivity quickly, set Q_D to 500 mL/min initially, run for 5 minutes until conductivity stabilizes, then set at 100 mL/min
Fresenius 4008E/H	≥300	No adjustment needed
	<300	Possible with use of an external flow meter and additional tubing to create a bypass
Fresenius 4008K	≥300	No adjustment needed
	100	No adjustment needed
Fresenius 4008S ARrT Plus	≥300	No adjustment needed
	200	No adjustment needed
Fresenius Genius	≥300	No adjustment needed
	<300	No adjustment needed
Gambro 200S Ultra	≥300	No adjustment needed
	100	Run in hemofiltration mode, set Q_R at 100 mL/min
		Instead of infusing, run replacement fluid as dialysate in countercurrent fashion

Q_D, dialysate flow rate; Q_R, reinfusate flow rate.

Dialysate containing citric acid as buffer (CitriSate) is now commercially available in the United States. There has been one report of reduced extracorporeal circuit clotting with its use for IHD in the critical care setting; however, further study is warranted before its use can be recommended, particularly with hybrid therapies.

Replacement Fluid Flow Rate for SLEDD-f

The ability to achieve and maintain greater convective clearance of middle-molecular weight solutes has potentially important therapeutic implications in critically ill patients with acute kidney injury and inflammatory or septic states. In this context, the principally diffusive solute clearance during SLEDD may be perceived as a disadvantage of this modality with respect to CRRT. A convective component can be added to the therapy with the use of adjunctive hemofiltration (SLEDD-f). Online production of ultrapure fluid for reinfusion is similar to the process during hemodiafiltration in chronic dialysis. In hybrid therapies, SLEDD-f has been performed primarily with the Fresenius 4008S ARrT-Plus. Online-produced substitution fluid is not yet approved by the Food and Drug Administration in the United States, but the technique is widely used elsewhere.

A specific variant of hybrid therapies using convection that has been reported in the United States is AVVH. This technique uses prepared replacement fluid packaged in bags, with an infusion rate of 4000 mL/h (67 mL/min) for 9 hours.

Timing of Treatment

Hybrid therapies may be performed during the day or at night. The rationale for nocturnal programs includes unrestricted patient access for diagnostic and therapeutic procedures during the day, as well as greater availability of hemodialysis machines at night. Potential disadvantages are safety issues and the need for troubleshooting at a time when there are fewer staff members available. Daytime treatments are recommended during the early phases when establishing a new hybrid therapy program, until such time as medical and nursing personnel are familiar and comfortable with the procedures.

Miscellaneous

Water Considerations

When high-flux membranes are used for dialysis, significant backfiltration may occur such that, even if the absence of direct infusion, solute, and water movement from the dialysate into the patient occurs in significant amounts. Endotoxin in the dialysate is of specific concern, and backfiltration of such may potentially further aggravate proinflammatory processes already ongoing in critically ill patients. Although definitive evidence is lacking, the use of ultrapure water for dialysate is prudent for all online fluid-generating therapies. On the other hand, use of ultrapure water is obligatory for online production of replacement fluid in hybrid therapies using convection, such as SLEDD-f.

It is therefore mandatory for hybrid therapy programs to have an appropriate water-quality assurance program in place. Standard water treatment entails bedside tap water being passed through three membrane filters: (1) a 10- μm filter to remove granulates and large particles; (2) activated charcoal to adsorb carbon, chloramines, and organic contaminants; and (3) a 1-μm filter to remove small particles. The latter is particularly prone to bacterial contamination resulting from the removal of chloramines. Water is then treated by reverse osmosis. The final step is further purification by a two- (Fresenius) or three-step (Gambro) ultrafiltration process to produce ultrapure water ready for mixing with electrolyte and bicarbonate concentrate. Water produced during this process as well as water obtained from the tap pretreatment must undergo a regular schedule of chemical, microbiological, chlorine/chloramines, and endotoxin assessment. Such verification of water quality is a paramount safety feature of hybrid therapies.

Nutrition

Although albumin loss in the dialysate is minimal in patients treated with SLEDD, intradialytic amino acid losses are approximately 1 g/h, and cumulative losses may be substantial with prolonged therapy. Expert opinion recommends that enteral or parenteral diet prescription be augmented with protein 0.2 g/kg/day for the duration of therapy to offset these losses.

Suggesting readings

Clark JA, Schulman G, Golper TA. Safety and efficacy of regional citrate anticoagulation during 8-hour sustained low-efficiency dialysis. *Clin J Am Soc Nephrol*. 2008;3:736.

Finkel KW, Foringer JR. Safety of regional citrate anticoagulation for continuous sustained low efficiency dialysis (C-SLED) in critically ill patients. *Renal Fail*. 2005;27:541.

Fliser D, Kielstein JT. A single-pass batch dialysis system: an ideal dialysis method for the patient in intensive care with acute renal failure. *Curr Opin Crit Care*. 2004;10:483-8.

Gashti CN, Salcedo S, Robinson V, Rodby RA. Accelerated venovenous hemofiltration: early technical and clinical experience. *Am J Kidney Dis*. 2008;51:804.

Hall JA, Shaver MJ, Marshall MR, Golper TA. Daily 12-hour sustained low-efficiency hemodialysis (SLED): a nursing perspective. *Blood Purif*. 1999;17:36.

Kielstein JT, Kretschmer U, Ernst T, Hafer C, Bahr MJ, Haller H, Fliser D. Efficacy and cardiovascular tolerability of extended dialysis in critically ill patients: a randomized controlled study. *Am J Kidney Dis*. 2004;43:342.

Kumar V, Craig M, Depner T, Yeun J. Extended daily dialysis: a new approach to renal replacement therapy for acute renal failure in the intensive care unit. *Am J Kidney Dis*. 2000;36:294.

Kumar VA, Yeun JY, Depner TA, Don BR. Extended daily dialysis vs. continuous hemodialysis for ICU patients with acute renal failure: a two-year single center report. *Int J Artif Organs*. 2004;27:371.

Marshall MR, Golper TA, Shaver MJ, et al. Sustained low-efficiency dialysis for critically ill patients requiring renal replacement therapy. *Kidney Int*. 2001;60:777.

Marshall MR, Golper TA, Shaver MJ, et al. Urea kinetics during sustained low-efficiency dialysis in critically ill patients requiring renal replacement therapy. *Am J Kidney Dis*. 2002;39:556.

Marshall M, Ma T, Galler D, et al. Sustained low-efficiency daily diafiltration (SLEDD-f) for critically ill patients requiring renal replacement therapy: towards an adequate therapy. *Nephrol Dial Transplant*. 2004;19:877.

Morath C, Miftari N, Dikow R, et al. Sodium citrate anticoagulation during sustained low efficiency dialysis (SLED) in patients with acute renal failure and severely impaired liver function. *Nephrol Dial Transplant*. 2008;23:421.

Naka T, Baldwin I, Bellomo R, et al. Prolonged daily intermittent renal replacement therapy in ICU patients by ICU nurses and ICU physicians. *Int J Artif Organs*. 2004;27:380.

Schneider M, Liefeldt L, Slowinski T, et al. Citrate anticoagulation protocol for slow extended hemodialysis with the Genius dialysis system in acute renal failure. *Int J Artif Organs*. 2008;31:43.

Tu A, Ahmad S. Heparin-free hemodialysis with citrate-containing dialysate in intensive care patients. *Dial Transplant*. 2000;29:620.

Part 4

Organizational Issues

Chapter 26

The ICU Environment

Ayan Sen

In the United States, more than 4 million patients are admitted to an intensive care unit (ICU) each year, ICU-related spending approaches $80 billion annually, and one in five of all deaths occur in a hospitalization involving the ICU. ICUs consist of teams of dedicated professionals working 'round-the-clock using the latest technologies to save lives that otherwise would have been lost.

The ICU has been the hallmark of the modern hospital, having come into prominence during the past 30 years. During the 1850s, Florence Nightingale was the first to suggest that critically ill patients need specialized, separate care. The development of ICUs was preceded by postoperative recovery rooms after World War II. The polio epidemic and subsequent performance of tracheotomy in a Copenhagen hospital with manual ventilation led to establishment of separate areas in the hospital to care for such patients. The birth of the mechanical ventilator in the 1950s was a fillip to the creation of dedicated units with specialized care.

The first Consensus Conference on Critical Care Medicine led by the National Institutes of Health (NIH) in 1983 pointed out that clinical practice has led to expanded indications for admissions to critical care units. Because of the use of expensive resources, ICUs should, in general, be reserved for those patients with reversible medical conditions who have a "reasonable prospect of substantial recovery." With recent changes in the healthcare environment, efficient use of ICUs has become a priority. Hospitals are increasingly using multidisciplinary approaches, checklists, and telemedicine approaches, and making efforts to improve patient flow. ICU burden may increase during the next few decades with the increasing elderly population with an array of comorbidities.

Purpose of ICU Care

The role of the ICU consists of enhanced patient monitoring, organ support, and prevention of complications. The focus of patient care is multisystem/multiorgan under the guidance of physicians and nurses who are specially trained in resuscitation and have a multidisciplinary approach to patient care.

Monitoring

The ICU provides the optimal setting for close monitoring of physiological changes, enabling active, rapid intervention. Patients may have monitoring of the following vital signs:

- *Cardiovascular*: Heart rate; telemetry; blood pressure (noninvasive); continuous blood pressure through arterial lines; central venous pressures (through central lines); hemodynamic indices through noninvasive/minimally invasive pulse pressure variation (Flotrac), bioimpedance, bioreactance, esophageal Doppler, and so on; and invasive devices such as pulmonary artery catheter, intra-aortic balloon counterpulsation, and mechanical cardiac devices
- *Respiratory*: Respiratory rate, pulse oximetry, mechanical ventilator numbers/waveforms
- *Neurological*: Intracranial pressure, cerebral perfusion pressure, and so on
- Renal: Urine output, daily input/output, electrolytes
- Infection: Temperature

Data derived from the monitoring systems should be interpreted in the context of individual clinical problems and coupled with therapeutic approaches.

Organ Support

The ICU is the place where temporary organ support is provided to failing organs. It includes the following:

- *Neurological support*: Sedation, intracranial pressure-guided therapy
- *Respiratory support*: Mechanical ventilators, noninvasive ventilation, extracorporeal membrane oxygenation
- *Cardiovascular support*: Vasopressors, inotropes, mechanical circulatory devices
- *Renal support*: Continuous renal replacement therapy (CRRT), ultrafiltration, hemodialysis
- *Gastrointestinal system*: Enteral/parenteral nutrition support
- *Endocrine system*: Insulin infusions, steroid therapy
- *Infection*: Antibiotic therapy
- *Hematological system*: Transfusions/plasmapheresis

Prevention of Complications

Prevention of complications from the underlying disease process and iatrogenic harm is the sine qua non of ICU care. In terms of managing patient safety in the ICU, the complex and multidisciplinary nature of intensive care medicine renders it particularly susceptible to the occurrence of medical errors/harm to patients. The following strategies have good evidence in the literature to reduce harmful outcomes:

- Sedation vacation and appropriate medication use to prevent critical illness delirium and long-term neurocognitive impairment

- Ventilator strategies/bundles to promote lung-protecting ventilation and to reduce injury. This "ventilator bundle" includes four components: elevation of the head of the bed to between 30 degrees and 45 degrees, daily "sedative interruption" and daily assessment of readiness to extubate, peptic ulcer disease prophylaxis, and venous thromboembolism prophylaxis (unless contraindicated).
- KDIGO guidelines for management of acute kidney injury
- Antibiotic stewardship
- Central line insertion checklist
- Bar-coding medication administration system to prevent adverse drug events
- Deescalating Foley catheters, lines if not needed to reduce Catheter-associated urinary tract infections and catheter-associated bloodstream infections
- Restricted blood transfusion
- Early nutrition initiation
- Adequate glycemic control
- Early physical therapy and mobility
- Multidisciplinary rounds and checklists

Choosing Wisely, an initiative of the American Board of Internal Medicine, created with the goal of "promoting conversations between physicians and patients by helping patients choose care supported by evidence, and free from harm has the following expectations for ICU patients:

- Reduced ordering of chest films and blood work in patients
- Transfusion threshold to 7 g/dL and greater unless hemodynamically unstable/bleeding
- No TPN within 7 days of ICU admission unless indicated clinically
- Daily sedation interruptions, analgesics before anxiolytics
- Palliative options for end-of-life care and for avoiding artificial prolongation of life

ICU Organizational Structure

The ICU team consists of the following providers (Figure 26.1):

Intensivists: Usually board-certified in critical care through internal medicine, surgery, anesthesiology, emergency medicine, or neurology. In some smaller systems, hospitalists assist in patient management in the ICU. Tele-ICU may have telemedicine intensivists directing care.

ICU nurses: ICU nurses are the primary caregivers of the patient and specialize in administering life-saving and life-sustaining therapy under the guidance of the intensivist/consultant teams. They are the primary patient advocates at the bedside.

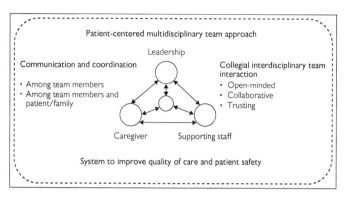

Figure 26.1 Four factors are needed to create an ideal intensive care unit (ICU) environment. A well-organized multidisciplinary approach can improve patient outcome.

ICU pharmacists: The ICU pharmacist usually makes rounds with the team and ensures appropriate choice of medications/reduction of adverse drug events, and compliance with pharmacy/ICU protocols.

Respiratory therapists: Experts in ventilator management, respiratory therapists also provide respiratory therapy such as nebulizer treatments, PEP therapy, and flutter valve and other forms of chest physical therapy.

Physical therapists/occupational therapists: Physical therapists in the ICU examine each individual and develop a plan using treatment techniques to promote the ability to move, reduce pain, restore function, and prevent disability. Occupational therapists are responsible for helping patients regain their ability to perform daily living and work activities.

ICU dietitians: Registered dietitians are qualified to evaluate the complex relationship between illness and malnutrition in the critically ill. They advocate for recommended feeding practices, bowel care, and so on.

Speech–language pathologists: The speech therapist evaluates and diagnoses speech, language, cognitive communication, and swallowing disorders.

Primary/consultant teams: ICU management involves a host of multiple specialties providing guidance in patient care. These teams may include cardiologists, nephrologists, hematologists, gastroenterologists, surgeons, palliative caregivers, neurologists, and so forth.

ICU mid-level practitioners: Consisting of physician assistants/nurse practitioners, these members assist the intensivist teams with patient management.

Case management nurses/social workers: Responsible for organizing a patient's case from admittance to discharge, a case management nurse understands hospital processes and the importance of making cost-effective decisions. Social workers in the ICU are uniquely qualified to assess and address many of the complex psychosocial circumstances that arise and can clarify potential misperceptions, enhancing communication among patients (if capacitated), their families, and the medical team members.

Vascular access specialists: These specialists assist in placement of ultrasound-guided peripherally inserted central lines, and radial arterial lines in some centers.

ICU clerks: ICU clerks ensure medical records, laboratory reports, radiological images, and other patient records are completed and secured properly, but are readily available. They have a critical role in ensuring optimal and safe patient care, and enabling medical and nursing staff members to do their work efficiently.

Pastoral care chaplains: Pastoral care chaplains focus on the spiritual well-being and support of patients and staff. They respond to emergency calls, deaths, and codes; make daily rounds in critical care units; and provide religious literature from various denominations as requested by the patient and/or family.

Additional support staff may be hired based on individual ICU needs and provisions (e.g., patient care assistants, specialized ECMO perfusionists in cardiothoracic ICUs, palliative nurse liaisons). Teamwork is the mantra in most ICUs, where each provider plays a valuable role in ensuring healing and provision of efficient and effective critical care.

ICU Models

ICUs can be "open" or "closed." Open units are those ICUs in which any physician in virtually any field may see a patient and write orders for that patient. Any physician may admit patients to these ICUs, with few limitations. Doctors are not required to obtain critical care consultations.

Closed ICUs are those in which physicians are required to admit patients to an intensive care service. Physicians must allow the ICU staff physicians to be the primary care agents for the patient, ultimately responsible for all medical decision making. Other disciplines may consult on the patient during the ICU stay. A collaborative model of ICU care is when the primary service admits patients to the ICU in consultation with the critical care service. Both services comanage patients. Reorganizing ICU physician services in one organization by implementing an intensivist infrastructure resulted in a 14% absolute risk reduction in mortality.

Tele-ICU

Tele-ICU refers to telemedicine technology in the care of ICU patients and has become a popular mode of critical care delivery. The tele-ICU team has access to all data elements related to patient care and can identify actual and potential issues related to patient care. High-resolution zoom cameras, microphones, and speakers are mounted in each ICU patient's room, providing the tele-ICU team one-way or two-way video/audio assessment capability and bedside communication. One model involves e-physicians making clinical determinations based on the data obtained from the telemonitors/electronic medical records (EMRs) and making decisions along with nurses at the bedside via virtual rounds. The physician is not at the bedside.

ICU telemedicine has significant potential to improve critical care delivery, but high-quality research is needed to inform its appropriate use best as a result of the high costs involved. The concept of a remote ICU team providing care remains foreign to some providers. Controversies and challenges will continue as tele-ICU programs grapple with reimbursement issues, cultural resistance, and interoperability of information technologies.

Types of ICUs

Different ICU models include the following:

- Mixed medical–surgical ICU
- Medical ICU
- Coronary care unit
- Surgical ICU
- Trauma ICU
- Neurological ICU
- Neurotrauma ICU
- Burn ICU
- Pediatric ICU
- Ob-Gyn ICU
- Neonatal ICU
- Abdominal transplant ICU

Challenges of the ICU Environment

The following challenges are imperative to the growth and sustainability of critical care departments and the delivery of efficient and effective critical care:

Clinical Challenges
- Operationalization of best evidence
- Admission/discharge criteria
- Team-based multidisciplinary care
- Patient safety
- Public health/disaster preparedness and ICUs
- Drug shortages
- Palliation and end-of-life care

Organizational Challenges
- Manpower and workforce
- Staffing models, nighttime intensivists, regionalization of critical care

- Models of ICU care: closed, open, collaborative
- Costs of care
- Financial challenges, pay-for-performance
- New healthcare reform and critical care medicine
- Growing and aging population
- Expensive care at the end of life
- Training in critical care
- Research and funding in critical care

Clinical Approach

A systematic approach to diagnosis and evaluation is necessary in the management of critically ill patients. When evaluating a new patient, the approach should include a primary survey, an AMPLE history, and a secondary survey:

- *Primary survey*: A, B, C, and D should be evaluated. A = protecting airway (neurological issues/respiratory issues), B = breathing (rate, pulse oximetry, work of breathing/use of accessory muscles), C = circulation (heart rate, blood pressure, clinical examination, hemodynamics if monitoring present), and D = neurological disability (e.g., Glasgow Coma Score, AVPU scale, National Institutes of Health Stroke Scale, CAM ICU score)
- *AMPLE*: The pneumonic stands for Allergies, Medications, Past medical history, Last meal, and Events leading to ICU admission
- *Secondary survey*: A head-to-toe examination should be performed. ICU management is dependent on attention to detail. Every clinical organ system should be assessed for abnormalities.

Clinical Presentation, Rounds, and Checklists

Presentation on rounds should include (1) a problem-based approach and management steps, and (2) a checklist of systems not covered in the problem-based approach. Usually the following systems-based issues are addressed: central nervous system (neurological); respiratory; cardiovascular; renal, fluids, and electrolytes; gastrointestinal and liver; hematological and coagulation issues; infection; endocrine issues; prophylaxis; lines and tubes; physical and occupational therapy goals; code status; and end-of-life care and family updates.

Some places use electronic/paper-based checklists that include aspects of critical care that may be missed. Using checklists during rounds has been shown to improve overall ICU outcomes. One such checklist uses the FASTHUGBID mnemonic:

F: Feeding
A: Analgesia
S: Sedation vacation attempted
T: Thromboprophylaxis
H: Head of bed elevation
U: Ulcer prevention
G: Glucose control
S: Spontaneous breathing trials
B: Bowel evaluation and maintenance
I: Indwelling catheter removal as soon as possible
D: Deescalation of antimicrobials and pharmacotherapies

Admission and Discharge Criteria

ICU admission criteria should be used to select patients who are likely to benefit from ICU care. Griner identified two conditions in which ICU care was of no greater benefit than conventional care: patients who are "too well to benefit" and patients who are "too sick to benefit" from critical care services. ICU care has been demonstrated to improve outcome in severely ill, unstable patient populations. Defining the "too well to benefit" and "too sick to benefit" population may be difficult based solely on diagnosis.

EMRs/Informatics Tools

The introduction of EMRs and computerized physician order entry into the ICU has transformed the way healthcare providers currently work. The challenge facing developers of EMRs is to create products that add value to systems of healthcare delivery. As EMRs become more prevalent, the potential challenges of safety and quality of care have increased. They have amplified cognitive overload and reduced situational awareness, leading to increased incidence of medical errors. New products such as AWARE are being used to improve signal-to-noise ratio when it comes to data from the ICU patient. (Developed at the Mayo Clinic in Rochester, AWARE is an Internet-based application that extracts data relevant to the treatment of critically ill patients and presents them to the provider in a systems-based package that provides dashboard visualization of organ system trends.) Challenges and opportunities lie in proving the value of health information systems. The future is likely to include better decision support systems, and use of the tools of computational biology and genomics to identify patterns in the clinical presentation of critical illness and to develop tailored therapy. Clinical trial recruitment using EMRs is also in the pipeline as exemplified by IBM Watson's collaboration with the Mayo Clinic, which uses cognitive computing capabilities to accelerate research and improve patient care.

ICU Design and Environmental Aspects

The concept of environmental influences on healing has been known since Florence Nightingale. The term *critical care unit* invokes images of very ill patients surrounded by the latest in biomedical equipment, monitoring devices, and code carts. These images alone can raise feelings of anxiety and levels of stress in patients and families. New generations of critical care units are being designed to promote healing in a humanistic manner that meets the holistic needs of patients and their families.

The following environmental aspects have been described to benefit healing and holistic critical care:

- Reduce environmental noise
- Provide adequate lighting
- Improve air quality and reduce offensive odors
- Provide hand-washing, hygiene, and toilet facilities
- Provide lifting devices
- Equip single rooms with televisions
- Implement open/unrestricted family visitation
- Provide family sleep rooms
- Incorporate nature/artwork in rooms
- Enable recreational therapy (e.g., music therapy, bedside art, pet therapy)
- Provide adequate transportation paths for patients
- Provide adequate material management, housekeeping functions, and storage facilities

Most healthcare providers have little experience designing and constructing an ICU. ICU design is complex and should include both clinically oriented and design-based multiprofessional team members. A design based on the functional requirements of the critical care unit and the consensus opinion of experts should enhance patient, family, and staff satisfaction and, in doing so, help protect the institution's bottom line.

ICU Outcome Measures

Clinical ICU outcome measures are important for research and quality control. Clinically meaningful outcomes measure how patients feel, function, and survive (e.g., mortality, quality of life). The National Quality Forum in the United States has endorsed measures of ICU outcomes (risk-adjusted mortality and length of stay) for public reporting. However, a large study of ICU patients in California found that public reporting of patient outcomes did not reduce mortality, but did result in reduced admission of the sickest patients to the ICU and increased transfer of critically ill patients to other hospitals. Other measures such as ICU mortality, hospital mortality, 90-day mortality, and 1-year functional outcome have been used, but they all have their pros and cons. The four major ICU predictive scoring systems are the Acute Physiologic and Chronic Health Evaluation (APACHE) scoring system, the Simplified Acute Physiologic Score (SAPS), the Mortality Prediction Model, and the Sequential Organ Failure Assessment (SOFA). A systemic review of the SOFA, SAPS II, APACHE II, and APACHE III scoring systems found the APACHE systems were slightly superior to the SAPS II and SOFA systems in predicting ICU mortality.

CRRT in the ICU

Intermittent hemodialysis is usually started, monitored, and completed by a dialysis nurse in the ICU. Sustained, low-efficiency dialysis may require the dialysis nurse to start therapy, change tubing, and so on, when there is a problem, and troubleshoot with alarms. The ICU nurse monitors therapy, and alerts the nephrologist and dialysis nurse about alarms and problems. CRRT is initiated, monitored, and managed by the ICU nurse. Policies and procedures are the responsibility of ICU nurse management in conjunction with nephrologists and intensivists.

No universal competencies exist for a CRRT program. Each facility develops its own education program and troubleshooting mechanisms. Policies and procedures are developed by nurse managers involved with the therapy. A good resource is available from the American Nephrology Nurses Association: *Continuous Renal Replacement Nephrology Nursing Guidelines for Care*. Furthermore, the manufacturers of the machines have education material and competency evaluations specific to the therapies they offer (NxStage, Prisma, and Fresenius [Fresenius Medical Care, Waltham, MA]).

The issue of who should manage CRRT in the ICU remains controversial in the absence of randomized controlled studies. Models of care include the intensivist or the nephrologist or both comanaging CRRT protocols. A combined approach is necessary for optimal patient outcome.

Key References

Angus DC, et al. Use of intensive care at the end of life in the United States: an epidemiologic study. *Crit Care Med*. 2004;32(3):638–643.

Angus DC, et al. Choosing wisely in critical care: maximizing value in the ICU. *Chest*. 2014;146(5):1142–1144.

Bellomo R, et al. Who should manage CRRT in the ICU? The intensivist's viewpoint. *Am J Kidney Dis*. 1997;30(5 suppl 4):S109–S111.

Griner PF. Treatment of acute pulmonary edema: conventional or intensive care? *Ann Intern Med*. 1972;77(4):501–506.

Halpern NA, Pastores SM. Critical care medicine in the United States 2000–2005: an analysis of bed numbers, occupancy rates, payer mix, and costs. *Crit Care Med*. 2010;38(1):65–71.

Kahn JM. The use and misuse of ICU telemedicine. *JAMA*. 2011;305(21):2227–2228.

Kellum JA, Lameire N. Diagnosis, evaluation, and management of acute kidney injury: a KDIGO summary (part 1). *Crit Care*. 2013;17(1):204.

Kollef MH, Schuster DP. Predicting intensive care unit outcome with scoring systems: underlying concepts and principles. *Crit Care Clin*. 1994;10(1):1–18.

Pronovost P, BS. A practical guide to measuring performance in the intensive care unit. *VHA Research Series*. 2002;2(29).

Vincent JL, et al. Thirty years of critical care medicine. *Crit Care*. 2010;14(3):311.

Chapter 27

Patient Care Quality and Teamwork

Kimberly Whiteman and Frederick J. Tasota

Quality patient care with successful outcomes depends on effective care delivery and requires an interprofessional approach to support a continuous renal replacement therapy (CRRT) program. To that end, the Acute Dialysis Quality Initiative was established in 2000 and continues to provide direction for the appropriate medical management of complicated patients with acute kidney injury by

- Establishing evidence-based statements
- Promoting consensus related to best practice
- Standardizing treatments for critically ill patients
- Facilitating research

Recommendations for determining the quality of CRRT delivered are not definitive in the literature; healthcare team members involved in the provision of direct patient care need to consider how quality care is best accomplished. The three components of Donabedian's classic model of quality health care (structure, process, and outcome) can be used to conceptualize the complex environment in which the care of patients on CRRT occurs (Figure 27.1).

Structure

Structure encompasses the characteristics of the healthcare providers and the physical and organizational setting where care is delivered. At the core of the CRRT interprofessional team are the renal physicians, intensivists, and intensive care unit (ICU) nurses. Other members may include pharmacists, nurse practitioners, physician assistants, and nursing leadership.

- *Characteristics of the healthcare providers* include their educational preparation to deliver quality care to patients with CRRT. Adequate didactic learning and hands-on training for nurses are critical. Physicians with expertise in different disciplines, including renal and critical care medicine, must also be educated to manage patients on CRRT. For most members of the team,

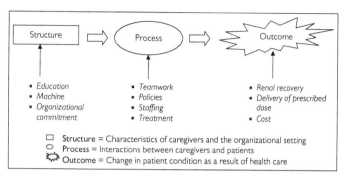

Figure 27.1 Donabedian model of quality health care adapted for continuous renal replacement therapy.

the addition of a CRRT program to the hospital requires the integration of a significant repertoire of knowledge and clinical skills. Other team members might include admitting physicians and a pharmacist. Finally, family and patient education materials should be developed to provide basic information to the recipients of care and their families.

- *The physical setting* is the actual patient care area where the treatments are prepared and delivered. Availability of sinks, water supply, and dialysis drains are a consideration in the selection of CRRT equipment. The physical setting in the pharmacy may be a determinant of whether to compound or purchase commercially prepared dialysate and replacement bags. Plans for cleaning and storage of machines when not in use, and adequate space for disposable supplies such as circuit and filter kits should be considered before starting a program.
- *Machines selected for treatment*, their advantages, and limitations are a part of the structure of a CRRT program. Products currently on the market vary with regard to the types of treatment that can be prescribed. Company specifications for the machines, available from the manufacturer, determine accuracy and capacity of pumps and scales.
- *Organizational commitment* to a CRRT program is necessary during startup to provide monies for machines, supplies, training, support services, and education. Routine and evolving needs, such as machine maintenance or replacement, require continued resource allocation to sustain the program. Organizations also need to commit to coordinate multiple hospital departments to expedite care. A CRRT program affects pharmacy, laboratory, central supply, and housekeeping departments. For instance, whether the hospital chooses to have pharmacy compound the replacement fluids or dispense a commercially prepared solution, the workload of the pharmacy will increase with each additional patient receiving treatment.

Process

Process in Donabedian's model is defined as the interactions among healthcare providers themselves and between healthcare workers and patients. Successful CRRT programs require collaboration and interprofessional teamwork, especially among the renal and intensive care physicians and the ICU nurses. CRRT policies and procedures, staffing, and treatment selection are processes that affect quality care.

- *Teamwork and collaboration* can be achieved through open communication. Forming an interprofessional CRRT team with members including a renal and intensive care physician, CRRT nurse educator, ICU manager, staff nurse, and pharmacist can help to encourage collaboration and teamwork. Ad hoc members can be included as needed. As the program evolves, the members can then use meeting times to share information and solve problems. Process improvement, quality, and safety issues can be addressed as a team.
- *Policies and procedures* should be in place to guide practitioners. Some suggestions for policies include the following:
  - Initiation, maintenance, and termination of treatment policies should be based on evidence. Evidence-based guidelines can be adapted to the local environment based on published procedures from professional organizations, such as the American Association of Critical Care Nurses or the American Association of Nephrology Nurses.
  - Accountability for patient care between renal dialysis and ICU nurses varies among practice settings. Some centers have renal dialysis nurses responsible for machine priming, initiating, and terminating treatment. In this model of care, the ICU nurse maintains the treatment, completes the intake and output, and performs basic troubleshooting. The renal dialysis nurse is available for troubleshooting more complicated problems. Other centers opt to have the ICU bedside nurse assume total responsibility for care related to CRRT. For this reason, careful delineation of roles needs to be determined before to the start of a program and evaluated periodically.
  - Documentation requirements, especially accurate documentation of intake and output, are a vital aspect of CRRT patient care. Charting models range from extensive flow sheets to a simplistic model of documenting only machine and catheter pressures and the amount of fluid removed from the patient.
  - Electronic medical record programmers need to understand how the CRRT machine calculates fluid balance to ensure accurate accounting of fluids. Double entry of fluids can occur when replacement or fluid volumes subtracted automatically by the CRRT machine are recorded as intake, or when effluent subtracted automatically by the machine are recorded as output.

- Fluids, medications, and laboratory tests appropriate only during the treatment need to be discontinued when CRRT is stopped. For instance, replacement fluid remaining on the medication administration record administered after CRRT is discontinued can quickly cause problems with fluid overload. Anticoagulation orders aimed at increasing filter life and routine CRRT laboratory tests should also be discontinued.
- Management of emergency situations should be planned before beginning a program. During a cardiac arrest, some centers routinely turn the net ultrafiltration rate to zero but continue blood circulation through the system. Others routinely return the blood if time permits, clamp all the lines, and discontinue treatment. The plan for management of emergencies needs to be determined by the interprofessional team and written into local policy.
- Physician accountability for writing CRRT orders should be determined by the physician groups and communicated clearly to the nursing staff and pharmacy. Consider who is responsible for the following:
  - Writing initial, daily, and discontinuation of CRRT orders
  - Inserting a temporary dialysis catheter and ensuring placement
  - Making changes to the orders based on changes in patient condition
- Responsibility for cleaning and storage of machines between patients is an important process to have in place. Centers for Disease Control and Prevention guidelines, hospital-specific infection control, and manufacturer recommendations should be used to write a policy for cleaning of equipment between patients.
- *Staffing and nursing care demands* created by a critically ill patient on CRRT can sometimes be daunting. Therefore, staffing requirements and assignments should, ultimately, be determined by the patient's condition and the skills of the available nursing staff. Consider 1:1 nurse-to-patient ratios for inexperienced CRRT nurses. As with any new skill, nurses who are unfamiliar with a procedure require more support and time than experienced nurses. The workload of the bedside nurse and, for many centers, the renal dialysis nurse increases with the initiation of a CRRT program. Consider who will assume responsibility for the following tasks:
  - Setup, priming, and takedown of circuits and/or machines
  - Initiation and termination of treatment
  - Patient monitoring during treatments
  - Troubleshooting at the bedside
  - Emergency procedures for rapid termination of treatment
- *Treatments* prescribed and processes chosen for obtaining supplies, dialysate, and replacement fluids affect care and staffing needs. Treatments that use anticoagulation protocols, such as heparin and citrate, may require more extensive monitoring of patients and laboratory results than treatments without anticoagulation. However, treatments provided with no

anticoagulation may also be associated with increased incidence of clotting and frequent filter changes that impact nursing time. Clinical choices should make sense for the patient and the organization, with quality patient care central to decision making.

Outcomes

Program outcomes of a positive nature are the result of careful delivery of CRRT interprofessional care. The ultimate goal of therapy is to have a complete recovery of renal function with no residual damage. To achieve this outcome, it is necessary not only to deliver care based on the best currently available evidence, but also to ensure the care is delivered as planned. Program outcomes and sustainability are dependent on delivery of the prescribed treatment at a reasonable cost.

Monitoring Quality

Monitoring quality is a vital aspect of any CRRT program. An interprofessional team model can be used to monitor and evaluate care delivery and facilitate implementing changes in practice when required. Initiatives should be directed toward each of the three components of quality healthcare: structure, process, and outcomes. Suggestions for monitoring the quality of care include the following activities:

- *Structure*: To provide quality care, the organization needs to have systems in place that support the CRRT program. The systems should be evaluated to be sure they are providing the level of support required by patients and staff. Some suggestions for evaluating the structure of CRRT care are as follows:
  - Educational programming evaluation. including attendance, course evaluations, posttest scores, or performance in CRRT simulation
  - Ongoing clinical competency programs for essential skills or to review high-risk/low-incidence problems systematically
  - Machine use, repair, and maintenance reviewed for patterns
  - History of alarm conditions to give insight into issues with care
  - Recommendations for classes, educational materials, and clinical competency programs obtained through trends in the literature, clinical experiences, or risk management reports
  - Effectiveness of programs to disseminate new information or a practice change to include whether the information is
    - Getting to the proper people
    - Being implemented into practice
    - Resulting in the expected clinical outcome

- *Process*: The interprofessional team should assess whether the policies and processes put in place to care for patients are followed. If the team determines processes are not being followed, the team should work with the nursing and medical staff to determine barriers and possible solutions. Considerations related to the process of care for patients on CRRT include the following:
  - Determine knowledge of and/or compliance with policies and procedures.
  - Provide periodic clinical updates relating to skills that are seldom performed.
  - Use machine alarm histories or a summary of calls to clinical support to provide information related to gaps in caregiver knowledge that may need to be addressed.
  - Audit the accuracy of documentation.
  - Standardize care as much as possible, including order sets or standardized processes to minimize the chance of error.
  - Collaborate with the pharmacy to determine the types of fluids being ordered and standardize prepared bags.
  - Complete root cause analysis or use other critical thinking tools to review process failures, identify solutions, and mitigate system problems.
- *Outcomes*: The interprofessional team should determine metrics to evaluate achievement of desired program outcomes. Some suggested metrics include the following:

  - Renal recovery rates measured and benchmarked against published rates for similar patients is a program outcome measurement. Review of case studies within the program or root cause analysis of identified problems can be used for program improvement.
  - Prescribed dose of CRRT compared with the actual delivered dose and achievement of fluid goals can be monitored. The team can identify frequently occurring reasons for not achieving the dose or fluid goals and can make practice changes for improvement.
  - The number of hours on treatment in a 24-hour period has several implications as a measure of quality. One measure uses the filter and circuit life compared with the expected life for treatments with similar anticoagulation and fluid flow rates. The reason for routine circuit changes can give the team insight into clinical practice. For instance, if most of the circuit changes occur as a result of clotting, quality improvement efforts might be implemented that encourage careful monitoring of filter pressures to encourage changing the circuit before the filter is clotted. The team could also consider examining the reason for noncontinuous treatment and consider practice changes to mitigate the most common barriers.
  - The cost of CRRT treatment and patient outcomes compared with alternative therapies can be used to evaluate current and future directions of the CRRT program.

Conclusion

Caring for patients with CRRT is complex and requires the collaboration of a highly skilled interprofessional team. Care delivery can be addressed using the structure, process, and outcome components of quality care. The implementation of a successful CRRT program and continued vigilance in all aspects of related care provide an effective support to patients with acute kidney injury and facilitate optimal recovery of renal function.

Key References

Acute Dialysis Quality Initiative. Acute Dialysis Quality Initiative homepage. http://www.adqi.net/. Accessed November 30, 2014.

Boyle M, Baldwin I. Understanding the continuous renal replacement therapy circuit for acute renal failure support: A quality issue in the intensive care unit. *AACN Adv Crit Care.* 2010;21(4):367–375.

Donabedian A. The Quality of Care: How can it be assessed? *JAMA.* 1988;260(12):1743–1748.

Godden J, Spexarth F, Dahlgren M. Standardization of continuous renal-replacement therapy fluids using a commercial product. *Am J Health Syst Pharm AJHP.* 2012;69(9):786–793.

Graham P, Lischer E. Nursing issues in renal replacement therapy: Organization, manpower assessment, competency evaluation and quality improvement processes. *Semin Dial.* 2011;24(2):183–187.

James MT, Tonelli M. Financial aspects of renal replacement therapy in acute kidney injury. *Semin Dial.* 2011;24(2):215–219.

Kleger G, Fässler E. Can circuit lifetime be a quality indicator in continuous renal replacement therapy in the critically ill? *Int J Artif Organs.* 2010;33(3):139–146.

Kocjan M, Brunet FP. Seeking optimal renal replacement therapy delivery in intensive care units. *Nephrol Nurs J.* 2010;37(1):47–53.

Mottes T, Owens T, Niedner M, Juno J, Shanley T, Heung M. Improving delivery of continuous renal replacement therapy: impact of a simulation-based educational intervention. *Pediatr Crit Care Med.* 2013;14(8):747–754.

Oh HJ, Lee MJ, Kim CH, et al. The benefit of specialized team approaches in patients with acute kidney injury undergoing continuous renal replacement therapy: propensity score matched analysis. *Crit Care.* 2014;18(4):454–454.

Roeder V R., Atkins HN., Ryan MA, Harms HJ. Putting the "C" back into continuous renal replacement therapy. *Nephrol Nurs J.* 2013;40(6):509–516.

Saadulla L, Reeves WB, Irey B, Ghahramani N. Impact of computerized order entry and pre-mixed dialysis solutions for continuous veno-venous hemodiafiltration on selection of therapy for acute renal failure. *J Med Syst.* 2012;36(1):223–231.

Chapter 28

Organizational Aspects

Developing Policies and Procedures for
Continuous Renal Replacement Therapies

Jorge Cerdá

This chapter describes the necessary steps to develop and maintain a successful Continuous Renal Replacement (CRRT) program. When initiating a CRRT program, it is necessary to consider the indications of the procedure (Table 28.1). By consensus, most experts agree that in hemodynamically unstable patients with acute kidney injury (AKI) requiring renal replacement therapy (RRT), CRRT should be the preferred modality.

Please see Table 28.1.

When nephrologists are faced with a patient with severe AKI requiring renal replacement therapy, multiple complex aspects must be considered (See Table 28.2).

Implementing CRRT: Requirements for a Successful Program

Extensive experience indicates that, five items appear to be critical to success: (bulleted list follows)

1. Motivation and involvement of a physician leader (usually a nephrologist)
2. Motivation and involvement of nursing education
3. Educated nursing staff
4. Standardized protocols and orders
5. Continuing education with (re)certification.

The care team must include (bulleted list follows)

- Nurses (critical care and/or nephrology)
- Physicians (nephrology and critical care, other subspecialties)
- Pharmacists
- Nutritionists

Table 28.1 Indications for specific renal replacement therapies

Therapeutic Goal	Hemodynamics*	Preferred Therapy
Fluid removal	Stable	Intermittent isolated ultrafiltration
	Unstable	Slow continuous ultrafiltration
Urea clearance	Stable	Intermittent hemodialysis
	Unstable	CRRT
		Convection: CVVH
		Diffusion: CVVHD
		Both: CVVHDF
Severe hyperkalemia	Stable/unstable	Intermittent hemodialysis
Severe metabolic acidosis	Stable	Intermittent hemodialysis
	Unstable	CRRT
Severe hyperphosphatemia	Stable/unstable	CRRT
Brain edema	Unstable	CRRT

CRRT, continuous renal replacement therapy; CVVH, continuous venovenous hemofiltration; CVVHD, continuous venovenous hemodialysis; CVVHDF, continuous venovenous hemodiafiltration. *In general, stable patients are those who do not require vasopressor therapy.

Table 28.2 Considerations in renal replacement therapy for AKI

Consideration	Components	Varieties
Dialysis Modality		
	Intermittent Hemodialysis	Daily, Every other day, SLED
	Continuous renal replacement therapies	AV, VV
	Peritoneal dialysis	
Dialysis Biocompatibility	Membrane characteristics	
Dialyzer Performance		
	Efficiency	
	Flux	
Dialysis Delivery		
	Timing of initiation	Early, Late
	Intensity of dialysis	Prescription vs. Delivery
	Adequacy of dialysis	Dialysis dose
Fluid management		Ultrafiltration, fluid balance
	Daily fluid balance	
	Management of fluid overload	

Factors affecting the performance of the CRRT program include the following: (bulleted list follows)

- Clear delineation of nursing responsibilities (setup, initiation, monitoring, troubleshooting)
- Clear delineation of physician responsibilities and interaction
- Formal and continuous education
- Standardized and updated protocols

Continuous quality improvement and innovationNotes

Policies and procedures, and personal interactions, must clearly establish from the start of the program who is in control of the technique and its application, and who is authorized to write orders and modify patient management, in agreement with the other members of the patient care team. Who is in charge of the procedure varies widely across the world and across the different models of intensive care units (ICUs) (closed or open format)

When developing a new CRRT program, positive and negative forces interact and determine the success or failure of the program: (bulleted list follows)

Forces in the Development of a CRRT Program

- Driving forces
  - Previous positive experiences/outcomes
  - Key staff resources, "champions"
  - Administration and physician support
  - Improved patient outcome
  - Knowledgeable critical care and nephrology nurses
- Restraining forces

  - Negative patient outcomes
  - Unclear/unrealistic expectations
  - Control: Who is in charge?
  - Staff inertia: "Big ships" are sometimes harder to steer
  - Resource availability and costs
    - Personnel
    - Equipment

Driving Forces

Previous positive experiences and improvement in patient outcome facilitate the development of the program. A point person—generally a nephrologist—champions the idea and gathers enough nursing, physician, and administrative support. A knowledgeable group of critical care and nephrology nurses is essential.

Restraining Forces

Given the severity of disease of the patients involved, initial negative patient outcome is common and becomes a potential hindrance in the growth of the program. "Negative" outcomes are intimately associated with unclear or unrealistic expectations. Clear, general goals for the program, and evaluable goals for the individual patient frequently avoid this problem and facilitate quality assurance measurements. In particular, we have seen fledgling programs begin by treating the sickest patients with highest expected mortality. Outcomes in such cases are predictably poor, leading to negative staff impressions of the overall efficacy of therapy.

In large institutions, staff inertia is an important restraining force. Conversely, in smaller institutions, unavailability of personnel and equipment may interfere severely with the success of the program.

Multiple factors affect the development of a CRRT program: (bulleted list follows)

Factors That Affect the Development of a CRRT Program

- Hospital factors
- Patient factors
- Availability of resources
- Equipment decisions
- Staff education
- Quality improvement
- Hospital factors
  - Size and type
  - Nature of services provided
  - Number of
    - ICU beds
    - Patients with acute renal failure (ARF) in the ICU per year
    - Patients with ARF dialyzed in the ICU per year
  - Mission
  - Commitment of administration
  - Dialysis services
  - ICU staffing
  - Level of intensive care unit
- Resources available
  - ICU staff support
  - Nephrology staff support
  - Dedicated budget
  - ICU staff education, training, and support
- Equipment decisions

- Ease of use
- Accuracy of measures
- Affordability
- Clinical support versus technical support

Hospital Factors

The size and type of hospital, and the nature of the services provided have a clear impact on the program. Larger hospitals with an active surgical program including cardiac and vascular surgery are more likely to generate a greater number of critical patients in need of CRRT. The size of the ICU is generally related to the size of these programs and has an important impact on resource availability. In addition, regardless of the size of the hospital, its "mission" usually has an important bearing on the growth of the program, because it determines the commitment of administration to, at least, a trial of the technique.

Patient Factors

Before initiating the program, the team must measure the number of AKI cases in the ICU per year, and the number of patients dialyzed during that interval, and estimate the number of CRRT procedures per year. Previous experience demonstrates that to maintain a staff proficient in CRRT, it is necessary to treat a minimum of 8 to 10 patients annually, with gaps between procedures not longer than 8 weeks. Overall, at least 12 CRRT procedures should be performed per year, with each procedure lasting a minimum of 5 to 7 days.

Resources Available

A recent national survey in the United States showed that, although hemodialysis nurses perform 90% of acute intermittent hemodialysis (IHD), approximately 50% of the CRRT patients are cared for jointly by hemodialysis and ICU nurses. In 30% of the institutions, the ICU nurse alone performs CRRT. In the majority of institutions, available resources include ICU and nephrology staff support, and a dedicated budget. Initial education, training, and ongoing support are essential for resource development.

More recent international surveys show significant variation in the distribution of physician and nursing responsibilities, with almost exclusively critical care-driven models in Asia and Australia/New Zealand, mixed responsibility in Europe, and greater nephrology involvement in the United States.

Which nurses should be selected? The desirable nurses are the critical thinkers, the problem solvers, and those who enjoy a challenge. In general, these nurses see technology as a means to improve care and they are able to "think in action."

Equipment Decisions

The main factors to consider include ease of use and accuracy of measures. Although, at the start, less expensive, simple equipment may appear preferable, in the long-term, more reliable and accurate equipment may not only ensure success, but also may be less costly. Better blood pump systems and tubing, appropriate biocompatible membranes and access by using longer lasting filters, may result in savings that overcome the initial expense. Furthermore, more complex, less reliable equipment is more costly in terms of nursing personnel and, by requiring 1:1 nursing at all times, severely interferes with resource availability.

Moreover, at the time of purchase, a clear distinction must be made between clinical and technical support. Rapid-response clinical support by knowledgeable nurses is most desirable on a 24-hour-a-day, 7-days-a-week basis.

Staff Education

When available, nephrology nurses provide valuable education on dialysis and access management. For critical care nurses unfamiliar with procedures, such know-how will flatten an otherwise steep learning curve. ICU-based critical care nurse specialists are essential to the education of the ICU staff, by placing CRRT in the appropriate context of overall patient care. In addition, ICU-based education establishes an all-important "ownership" of the procedure. In a gradual fashion, ICU nurses learn that, rather than merely adding another piece of equipment to an already cluttered bedside, CRRT provides virtually complete control of nutrition, hemodynamics, fluid, electrolytes, and acid–base management that facilitates rather than complicates patient support.

Pharmacists must be part of the group from the start, and nutritionists must understand the new requirements of CRRT patients. Often, these patients have different, and sometimes opposite, needs to those of patients on IHD.

The success of a CRRT program is critically dependent on the performance of an ongoing quality improvement program: (bulleted list follows)

Quality Improvement

Quality Improvement: Components
• Staff
  • Education
  • Clinical support
  • Competency
• Patient
  • Early identification
  • Response to treatment
  • Untoward events
  • Vascular access
• System
  • Staffing
  • Supplies

- Equipment
- Outcome
  - Patient goal achieved
  - Patient outcome
    - Survival
    - Renal function status
  - Staff satisfaction
  - Costs
  - Errors are unfortunately frequent, especially in the delivery of prescribed fluid balance and utilization of dialysis fluids: (bulleted list follows)

Sources of Fluid Balance and Dialysis Errors
- Inappropriate prescription
- Operator error
- Machine error
- Recommendations to prevent complications and errors include: (bulleted list follows)

Recommendations for Preventing Complications during Ultrafiltration with Hybrid/CRRT Modalities
- All operators of intermittent or continuous renal replacement machines should be trained appropriately and certified initially and on a periodic basis.
- All operators of such machines must be aware of the potential complications of overriding machine alarms.
- Intensive care and dialysis units should record hourly and total effluent volumes during CRRT, and pre- and posttreatment weights and ultrafiltration loss for intermittent therapies

When a new procedure is initiated, it is necessary to evaluate the process and its outcomes. The major question is: Does this therapy make a difference? The improvement process begins at the inception of the program and examines staff, patient, and system issues as well as clinical outcomes. Staff education, clinical support, and competency should be ongoing. Patient outcomes are measured in three domains: achievement of goal of therapy, patient survival, and preservation of renal function. Outcome evaluation must include staff satisfaction. System and financial concerns are also monitored. Analysis of data includes periodic revision of orders, flow sheets, protocols, education, filters and circuits, anticoagulation, and equipment.

Role of the Nephrologist

Nephrologists who treat critically ill patients with ARF must change from having a focused role to a more global role in terms of patient care. By their ability to achieve continuous, effective metabolic, fluid, and electrolyte control, nephrologists in charge of CRRT must interact continuously and come to a consensus with all the other practitioners involved. These nephrologists must have a solid presence in the ICU, be knowledgeable of the problems affecting their patients, and become part of the team—a recognizable presence who solves problems reliably and is seen by ICU staff as a relevant practitioner in that environment.

Nephrologists participate in modality and equipment decisions, fluid management (volume and composition), and dose of dialysis prescription, anticoagulation, nutrition, and drug adjustment in continuous collaboration with the other members of the patient care team. Moreover, nephrologists are key in making decisions on treatment initiation and discontinuation. Continuous measurement of severity of disease by widely accepted scoring systems is desirable to evaluate patient outcomes and quality assurance.

In this important field of medicine, where critical care and nephrology overlap, the size of the practice and the scope of knowledge is so wide that the evolution of a new subspecialty, Critical Care Nephrology, is justified (see Chapter 26).

Financial Considerations

Characteristics of the "Ideal" Treatment Modality of ARF in the ICU
- Preserves homeostasis
- Does not increase comorbidity
- Does not worsen patient's underlying condition
- Is inexpensive
- Is simple to manage
- Is not burdensome to the ICU staff
- Cost is an important consideration. Multiple assessments of the cost of renal replacement therapy for ARF suggest that CRRT is more expensive than IHD. However, cost considerations depend on what is included: (bulleted list follows)

Is CRRT More Expensive Than IHD? It Depends on What You Count
- Use of personnel
  - One-to-one versus 1:2 nursing; dialysis nurses involved?
- Equipment
  - Initial expense: type of machine
  - Filter life
  - Replacement and dialysis fluids: pharmacy costs
- Lab costs
- Respirator days, ICU length of stay

Other Modifiers of Cost
- Predetermined changes of the extracorporeal circuit
  - Scheduled changes

- Minimal filtrate to blood urea nitrogen concentration (FUN/BUN)ratio (generally 0.8)
- Anticoagulation
  - Filter survival
  - Replacement solutions
  - Labs
- Cost increases when higher amounts of therapy are delivered:
  - IHD: personnel costs increase
  - CRRT: replacement solutions and dialysate

Areas of Potential Cost Reduction in CRRT

- Filters
  - Type of membrane
  - Access (a major factor)
  - Anticoagulation (a major factor)
- Personnel
  - ICU nursing alone versus nephrology and critical care nursing collaboration
- Dialysate and replacement fluids
- Service, support
- Appropriateness of treatment, patient selection

Several recent articles suggest CRRT is superior to IHD with respect to renal recovery. Implications go far beyond just the "hard" end point of renal recovery: (bulleted list follows)

- The need for chronic dialysis impairs quality of life.
- If the ICU stay can be reduced, it will have a major impact on the hospital budget.
- Patient dependent on chronic dialysis consumes significant healthcare resources and affects the community healthcare budget.

Key References

Bellomo R, Cole L, Reeves J, Silvester W. Renal replacement therapy in the ICU: the Australian experience. *Am J Kidney Dis*. 1997(5 suppl 4):S80–S83.

Clark WR, Letteri JJ, Uchino S, Bellomo R, Ronco C. Recent clinical advances in the management of critically ill patients with acute renal failure. *Blood Purif*. 2006;24(5–6):487–498.

Kellum JA, Cerda J, Kaplan LJ, Nadim MK, Palevsky PM. Fluids for the prevention and management of acute kidney injury. *Int J Artif Organs*. 2008;31: 96–110.

Martin RK, Jurschak J. Nursing management of continuous renal replacement therapy. *Semin Dial*. 1996;9(2):192–199.

Mehta RL, Lettieri JM, the National Kidney Foundation Council on Dialysis. Current status of renal replacement therapy for acute renal failure: a survey of US nephrologists. *Am J Nephrol*. 1999;19:377–382.

Mehta RL, Martin RL. Initiating and implementing a continuous renal replacement therapy program. *Semin Dial*. 1996;9(2):80–87.

Monson P, Mehta RL. Nutritional considerations in continuous renal replacement therapies. *Semin Dial*. 1996;9:152–160.

Paganini EM, Tapolyai M, Goormastic M, et al. Establishing a dialysis therapy/patient outcome link in intensive care unit acute dialysis for patients with acute renal failure. *Am J Kidney Dis*. 1996;28(5 suppl 3):S81–S89.

Silvester W, Bellomo R, Cole L. Epidemiology, management, and outcome of severe acute renal failure of critical illness in Australia. *Crit Care Med*. 2001;29(10):1910–1915.

Uchino S, Bellomo R, Morimatsu H, et al. Continuous renal replacement therapy: a worldwide survey. *Intensive Care Med*. 2007;33(9):1563–1570.

Chapter 29

Documentation, Billing, and Reimbursement for Continuous Renal Replacement Therapy

Kevin W. Finkel

Billing Codes

Initial Inpatient Consultations—New or Established Patients (CPT Codes 99251–99255)

New or established hospitalized patients who are seen for an initial consultation are billed under the Current Procedural Terminology (CPT) codes 99251 to 99255. To meet the requirements for proper documentation, there must be a written request for the consultation, and the results of the consultation must be made available to the requesting physician. This requirement is easily met with either a written or dictated note in the inpatient medical record.

The level of service billed (level 5 being highest) is based on the complexity of the particular patient supported by the appropriate documentation. It is likely that most, if not all, patients in the intensive care unit (ICU) who require continuous renal replacement therapy (CRRT) will be ill enough to justify a level 5 visit.

There are three components to medical documentation: the history, physical examination, and decision making. For a level 5 initial consultation, all three components must be detailed and medically complex. Documentation for a level 5 consultation requires a *comprehensive history* (chief complaint, four elements of the history of the current illness, a 10-point review of systems, and complete past, family, and social histories), a *comprehensive physical examination* (vital signs plus examination of eight organ systems), and *highly complex decision making* (extensive number of diagnoses or treatment options, complex data, and high risk of morbity and/or mortality to the patient).

Consultation codes (99521–99255) have been eliminated by Medicare. Instead, they have been replaced with the initial inpatient codes (99221–99223). Several commercial payers, however, still reimburse for consultation codes. Therefore, it is prudent to check with your local providers for specific information (Box 29.1).

Initial Hospital Care for a New or Established Patient (CPT Codes 99221–99223)

If a patient is admitted under the direct care of the physician who will also provide CRRT, then the initial evaluation can be billed under CPT codes 99221 to 99223. The level of service billed (level 3 being the highest) is based on the complexity of the particular patient supported by the appropriate documentation. It is likely that most, if not all, patients admitted to the ICU will be ill enough to justify a level 3 visit. As with a level 5 initial consultation, documentation requires a comprehensive history and physical examination, and complex decision making with an extensive number of diagnoses or treatment options, complex data, and high risk to the patient.

Critical Care Services (CPT codes 99291–99292)

Initial and subsequent care of the critically ill patient may be billed with the critical care services CPT codes 99291 and 99292. Such patients should be critically ill, usually with multiple-organ dysfunction syndrome. Documentation must state explicitly that the patient is critically ill, and it should include such factors as the degree of hemodynamic instability and its treatment. The mere fact that a patient is situated in the ICU is not sufficient justification for billing critical care services. Critical care service is a time-dependent CPT code: the first 30 to 74 minutes of critical care is billed as 99291; the code 99292 is used for each additional 30 minutes. The total critical care time must be documented in the medical record. Multiple physicians may bill for critical care if the services involve multiple organ systems (unrelated diagnoses), but the actual period of billing cannot overlap, so it is best to document the actual time periods spent at the patient's bedside. Also, no more than a total of 3 hours of critical care time can be billed in a single 24-hour period.

Continuous Dialysis/CRRT (CPT Codes 90945 and 90947)

CRRT can be billed for on the initial day of patient encounter and subsequent days with the CPT codes 90945 and 90947 (*procedure other than hemodialysis* [*e.g., peritoneal, hemofiltration*]). To bill for continuous dialysis, it must be clearly stated in the medical record that the patient was seen during dialysis.

Code 90945 (*procedure other than hemodialysis* [*e.g., peritoneal, hemofiltration*] *with single-physician evaluation*) is billed if only one visit is required. However, ICU patients usually require multiple reassessments throughout the day. Regardless of whether there is a change in the dialysis prescription, as long as there is appropriate documentation of the need for multiple assessments, then 90947 (*procedure other than hemodialysis requiring repeated evaluations, with or without substantial revision of the dialysis prescription*) can be billed. The medical record should include such factors as the degree of hemodynamic instability, changes in acid–base status, and change in replacement fluid. Documentation of the degree of hemodynamic instability is necessary to be reimbursed properly for CRRT procedures. When more than one visit to the bedside is needed, it is appropriate to bill 90947.

Subsequent Hospital Follow-up (CPT Codes 99231–99233)

CPT codes 99231 to 99233 are used to bill for subsequent hospital follow-ups. Most critically ill patients will qualify for a level 3 (highest severity) service. Documentation for a level 3 follow-up requires that two of the three components of the chart note be detailed. This requirement is most commonly met with a *detailed physical examination* (vital signs plus examination of five to seven organ systems) and *highly complex decision making*.

Dialysis Catheters and Modifiers for Multiple Procedures

Placement of temporary dialysis catheters (CPT code 36556) can be billed at any time. It is billed with a 25 modifier linked to the evaluation and management (E&M) CPT code billed the same day (initial or follow-up codes). For example, if a patient is billed for subsequent hospital follow-up (99233) and a dialysis catheter is also placed on that day, then 99233.25 and 36556 are billed. The 25 modifier is linked to the E&M code and signifies there is *a significant and separately identifiable procedure*.

When multiple procedures are done on the same day, then a 51 modifier is also used. The 51 modifier is linked to all procedures after the first. For example, on the initial hospital day, if a physician performs a consultation, places a temporary dialysis catheter, and sees the patient after CRRT is initiated, then all three encounters can be billed: 99255.25 (initial consult with a significant and separately identifiable procedure), 36556 (placement of a temporary dialysis catheter), and 90945.51 (CRRT with multiple procedures).

Initial Patient Evaluation

The initial evaluation of a patient in the ICU by a consultant can be billed by CPT codes 99251 to 99255 or 99221 to 99223 (depending on the insurance provider) based on the complexity of the particular patient supported by the appropriate documentation. If, on the day of consultation, CRRT is performed, and the consultant is present for a portion of the CRRT procedure, then a bill for CRRT (90945 or 90947) can also be charged with a 25 modifier (*significant and separately identifiable procedure*). However, after the initial evaluation, subsequent dialysis days allow billing for only one CPT code (continuous dialysis or subsequent hospital follow-up) because E&M is built into dialysis codes.

If a patient is admitted to the physician who will also provide CRRT care, then CPT codes 99221 to 99223 (initial hospital care for a new or established patient) can be used along with CRRT codes (90945 or 90947) on the initial day with the appropriate documentation and the 25 modifier. As an alternative to the initial CPT codes for consultation or inpatient admission, a critical care code (99291–99292) may be used.

Subsequent Hospital Days

In the daily follow-up of patients on CRRT, CPT codes 90945 and 90947 are traditionally used. Because these codes (as opposed to other procedure codes) include an E&M component, it is improper to bill separately a follow-up (99231–99233) and a CRRT code. In all cases, after the initial day of evaluation, subsequent billing can only be a single CPT code, either CRRT or subsequent hospital follow-up. Per the guidelines of the Centers for Medicare and Medicaid Services (CMS), if both CRRT and another E&M service are billed on subsequent hospital days, then *pay only the dialysis service and deny any other evaluation and management service*. Choosing to bill for CRRT or subsequent follow-up is at the physician's discretion.

If critical care services are billed on subsequent hospital days, it is permissible to link the CRRT code using the 25 modifier. However, this should be done with extreme caution. To bill both subsequent critical care and CRRT, two totally separate, clearly identified patient encounters must be documented. It is hard to focus on critical illness without consideration of acid–base status, electrolyte abnormalities, and hemodynamic parameters without significant overlap with CRRT E&M.

Relative Value Units

The relative value unit (RVU) is the common scale by which practically all physician services are measured. CMS and most other insurers use RVUs to determine the reimbursement rate for services after incorporating geographic and other factors.

The resource-based relative value scale (RBRVS) assigns a relative value to each CPT code relative to all the other CPT codes. The RBRVS was developed for CMS and, in 1992, Medicare established its standardized physician payment schedule based on the RBRVS.

RVUs are determined by committees of the American Medical Association. The committee members come from all medical specialties and include representatives from other health professions, including nursing. The committee assigns a relative value after hearing testimony from specialty groups on how many hours or minutes it takes to perform a procedure, the level of skill required, the level of education/training required, and the practice expense associated with a procedure (Box 29.2).

There are three components to a relative value—practice expense (*PE*), work (*w*), and malpractice (*MP*). Each component is adjusted geographically using three separate geographic practice cost indexes (*GPCI*). This relative value is then multiplied by a single, nationally uniform "conversion factor" to arrive at a monetary value. The CMS conversion factor for 2015 is approximately 35.8. The payment formula is

$$Payment = [(wRVU \times wGPCI) + (PERVU \times MP\,GPCI)] \times CF,$$

where *CF* is the conversion factor.

Box 29.2 RVU Associated with Common CPT Codes

CPT Code	RVU
99255 (Initial consult)	4.0
99291 (Critical care 30–74 minutes)	4.5
99223 (Initial inpatient admission)	3.86
90945 (Single CRRT)	1.56
90947 (Repeat CRRT)	2.52

CPT, Current Procedural Terminology; CRRT, continuous renal replacement therapy; RVU, relative value unit.

Depending on the contract, insurers may pay at or above Medicare rates. Actual RVU levels are subject to change, but Box 29.2 lists those for common CPT codes.

Summary

- Thorough documentation and correct coding are essential for timely and appropriate reimbursement.
- New patients can be billed as initial inpatient consults, initial hospital care, or critical care services.
- If, on the day of consultation or admission, CRRT is performed, and the physician is present for a portion of the CRRT procedure, then a bill for CRRT can also be charged with a 25 modifier (significant and separately identifiable procedure).
- Multiple procedures can be billed with the 51 modifier attached to all procedures after the first.
- After the initial day of evaluation, subsequent billing can be a single CPT code only, either CRRT or subsequent hospital follow-up. CRRT can be billed daily using a 25 modifier with subsequent critical care codes; however, it is challenging to meet the documentation requirements for both encounters.
- Per the guidelines of CMS, if both CRRT and another E&M service are billed on subsequent hospital days, then *pay only the dialysis service and deny any other evaluation and management service* (excludes critical care).
- The RVU is the common scale by which practically all physician services are measured. CMS and most other insurers use RVUs to determine the reimbursement rate for services after incorporating geographic and other factors.
- The CMS conversion factor for 2013 is approximately 35.8.

Chapter 30

Machines for Continuous Renal Replacement Therapy

Claudio Ronco

In 1977, Peter Kramer introduced for the first time a simple therapy called *continuous arteriovenous hemofiltration* (CAVH). In the following years, CAVH represented an important alternative to hemodialysis or peritoneal dialysis, especially for those patients in whom severe clinical conditions precluded the traditional forms of renal replacement. CAVH enabled small centers not equipped with hemodialysis facilities to perform acute renal replacement therapy. The technique, however, displayed its limitations rapidly and, despite a good fluid control, urea clearance could not exceed 15 L every 24 hours. Because most critically ill patients are severely catabolic, the amount of urea removed frequently resulted in an insufficient control of blood urea levels and inadequate blood purification. For this reason, Geronemus and cowork-ers, in 1984, introduced the use of continuous arteriovenous hemodialysis (CVVHD). The treatment was similar to CAVH, but a low-permeability membrane could be used and countercurrent dialysate flow was provided to increase urea removal by the addition of diffusion. A daily urea clearance in the range of 24 to 26 L could be achieved with continuous arteriovenous hemodialysis. At that time, Ronco and colleagues applied the same concept to a highly permeable hollow fiber hemodiafilter, and first described the treat-ment called *continuous arteriovenous hemodiafiltration* (CVVHDF). With that treatment, the high convection rates combined with the countercurrent dialy-sate flow allowed increased removal of small and large molecules.

One of the major limitations imposed by the arteriovenous approach was the unstable performance of the circuit resulting from possible reductions of extracorporeal blood flow secondary to the patient's hypotension, line kink-ing, and filter clotting. This often resulted in treatment interruptions, reduced daily clearance, and treatment failure. Initially, the use of continuous renal replacement therapy (CRRT) was limited to tertiary care centers, but over time, and by the late 1980s, CRRT had become more and more accepted in intensive care units (ICUs) as a standard form of therapy. A major advance was the introduction of machines that could perform continuous venove-nous hemofiltration (CVVH) or continuous venovenous hemodiafiltration (CVVHDF), which used a standard double-lumen dialysis catheter. As a con-sequence, the use of CAVH started to decline and the more efficient CVVH began to become preferred. CVVH can be performed in postdilution mode, reaching daily clearances for urea in the range of 36 to 48 L. When predilution is performed, the requirement of heparin may be remarkably reduced and ultrafiltration can be increased up to 48 to 70 L/24 h. Because predilution decreases the effective concentration of the solute in the ultrafiltered blood, the amount of solute removal is not proportional to the amount of ultrafiltration and it must be scaled down by a factor depending on the percent of predilution versus blood flow.

The increased amount of fluid exchanged per day in CVVH required automated blood modules equipped with blood leak detectors, pressure alarms, and pressure drop measurements in the dialyzer. However, despite the achievement of greater efficiency, safety, and reliability, there were still limitations because these machines were essentially derived from hemodialysis blood devices and were never designed as self-standing units for CRRT. In most cases, volumetric pumps were added to a blood module to achieve ultrafiltration and replacement fluid volume control. This approach is still in use in several units and it is defined as adaptive technology. Adaptive technology may be very effective, but it presents the risk of operating with components that are not interconnected, and therefore they are not completely safe according to the standards of an integrated machine. For this reason, a full spectrum of CRRT machines has evolved throughout the years to become safer, more reliable, and easier to use (Figure 30.1).

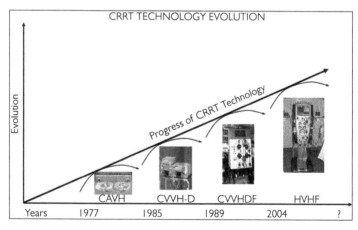

Figure 30.1 Evolution of CRRT techniques over the years with a continuous progress towards a more sophisticated technology.

Machines for CRRT

The modern history of CRRT is characterized by the development of complete CRRT machines designed specifically for acute renal replacement in ICU patients (Figure 30.2). These machines are all equipped with integrated safety alarms, fluid-balancing controls, and connected blood modules with the capability of performing CVVH, continuous venovenous hemodialysis (CVVHD), and CVVHDF. Such machines can now achieve a smooth conduction of the renal replacement treatment in the ICU and they can perform continuous as well as intermittent renal replacement therapies with increased levels of efficiency. Blood flows up to 500 mL/min and dialysate/replacement fluid flow rates of up to 200 to 300 mL/min are leading to urea clearances that may reach levels close to standard intermittent hemodialysis machines. At the same time, the highly permeable membranes used in CRRT systems achieve improved clearance of the larger molecular weight solutes. As a result of to the higher blood and dialysate flow rates achievable in the system, higher surface areas can now be used and more efficient treatments can be carried out. The fluid control is achieved via gravimetric or volumetric control systems that drive peristaltic pumps both for ultrafiltration and reinfusion. The priming procedures are simplified because of the step-by-step online help and the self-loading preassembled tubing sets.

The new machines are also equipped with a user-friendly interface, which leads to increased confidence in the personnel administering the therapy, and constant levels of efficiency can be obtained without major problems or complications. Some of the new machines present operational conditions similar to those used for chronic hemodialysis, which provides the possibility of using the machines for different treatments and purposes (Table 30.1). Most machines work either in a pure convection or diffusion or combined mode. Again, the most recent machines have the capability of performing treatments with high exchange volumes, such as high-volume hemofiltration. In these circumstances, the presence of an adequate warmer for the substitution fluid is very important to maintain thermal balance. In this field, online monitors for thermal balance and for blood volume determination are available on the market, but they are integrated in the machines in isolated cases only. New machines are equipped with preset disposable circuits or with easy instructions for the rinsing/priming phase of the therapy. The user-friendly interface plays an important role in the selection of the therapy mode and the smooth conduction of the entire session, which makes these machines well suited for use in ICUs, where the experience of the personnel may not be as wide as in the dialysis setting. The presence of an increased number of pressure sensors in the machines renders the monitoring of the treatment easier and accurate. In particular, the measurement of the end-to-end pressure drop in the filter allows for the monitoring of the patency of the blood compartment and allows the early identification of clotting or filter malfunction. In some machines, the pressure transducers are designed to prevent the contact of blood with air, and the lines are constructed with special membrane buttons that transmit the pressure values to the sensor without air-to-blood interface. The measurement of net ultrafiltration and the balance between ultrafiltration and reinfusion is done with one or two scales in different machines, or with volumetric fluid control. Most of these systems also operate in continuous hemodialysis to achieve the desired balance between the dialysate inlet and the dialysate outlet.

Metabolic control of acute renal failure generally requires at least 30 L urea clearance/day, and positive outcomes have considered adequate a dosage greater than 35 mL/kg/h, although some evidence may suggest that dosages between 20 mL/kg/h and 35 mL/kg/h can be equally safe. The combination of diffusion and convection has shown that satisfactory clearances of small and medium–large molecules can generally be achieved. Furthermore, in cases of sepsis, patients may present increased levels of substances in the middle-molecular weight range (500–5000 Da), such as chemical mediators of the humoral response to endotoxins. In this case, the treatment should control not only urea and other waste products, but also the circulating levels of these proinflammatory substances. To achieve such a complex task, high convective rates may be required. In these conditions, the necessary rate of convection can be obtained in continuous hemofiltration, in continuous hemodiafiltration (in this case, four pumps are required), or in continuous high-flux hemodialysis with continuous dialysate volume control (three pumps are required along with a reliable ultrafiltration control system). In hemodiafiltration, dialysate outlet flow exceeds the volume of inlet dialysate volume and the required ultrafiltration, and for this reason a replacement fluid is required. In high-flux hemodialysis, substitution fluid is not required and the balance is obtained by a mechanism of internal backfiltration. Warmed dialysate is delivered at a programmed flow rate and the second pump regulates the dialysate outlet flow rate and net ultrafiltration with a continuous volume control. In some machines, this treatment has been performed in recirculation mode and it has been defined *continuous high-flux hemodialysis* because of the internal filtration–backfiltration mechanism similar to that of high-flux hemodialysis in chronic hemodialysis. When the patient's dry weight has been achieved, the circuit may operate at zero net ultrafiltration using sterile dialysate at various flows (50–200 mL/min). With relatively high-volume hemofiltration (2–3 L/h), hemodiafiltration, or high-flux hemodialysis, the clearance of small and large molecules is improved. If performed continuously, the treatments can provide weekly Kt/V in the range of 7 to 10, resulting in treatment efficacy much greater than that achieved with other intermittent dialysis therapies. At the same time, significant amount of proinflammatory mediators can be removed, leading to improved hemodynamic stability.

Besides the number of the pumps, an important feature of CRRT machines is the operator interface. The wide color screen of some machines allows easy access to required information and online help for most of the functions. The issue of collecting the treatment data is an important one, and almost all machines

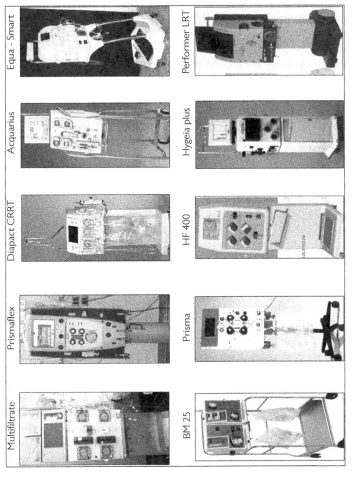

Figure 30.2 A group of CRRT machines developed in recent years.

Equa - Smart

Performer LRT

Acquarius

Hygeia plus

Diapact CRRT

HF 400

Prismaflex

Prisma

Multifiltrate

BM 25

Table 30.1 Characteristics of recent CRRT machines

	Company	Pumps	Qb (ml/min)	Qd (ml/min)	Fluid manag (Liters)	Heater	Heparin Pump	Reinfus sites	Pressure sensors	Printer/ RS-332 P	Scales	Possible techniques
Acquarius	Ew L S Baxter	4	0–450	0–165	10 L	Y	Y	Pre Post Pre-post	4	no Y	2	(IHD-IHFD)-IHF, PEX-PAP SCUF -CVVH - CVVHD- CVVHFD Pediatric Tx
BM 25	Ew L S Baxter	3	30–500	0–150	16 L	no	no	Pre Post	2	no Y	2	SCUF-CVVH-CVVHD-PEX Pediatric Tx (Qb=5-150 ml/min)
Diapact	B.Braun	3	10–500	5–400	25 L	Y	no	Pre Post	4	no Y	1	IHD-IHFD-IHF, PEX-PAP SCUF -CVVH - CVVHD-
Equa-Smart	Medicine	2*	5–400	0–150	10 L	Y	Y	Pre Post	3	Y Y	3	CVVHFD SCUF-CWH- CVVHD -CVVHDF- PEX - Pediatric Tx
2008 H 2008K	FMC-NA	1+3**	0–500	0–300	open	Y	Y	no	3	no Y	Volumetric	IHD-IHFD, SLED-SCUF-CVVHD Pediatric Tx
Multimat B	Bellco	2***	0–400	0–75	25 L	no	Y	Pre Post	3	no no	1	SCUF-CVVH-CVVHD-CPFA

HF = 400	Informed	4	0–450	0–200	12 L	Y	Y	Pre Post Pre-Post	4	no Y	2	IHD-IHFD-IHF, PEX, SCUF - CVVH - CVVHD - CVVHDF -Pediatric Tx
Hygeia plus	Kimal	4	0–500	0–66	4 L	Y	Y	Pre Post Pre-Post	4	Y Y	Volu-metric	SCUF-CVVH- CVVHD CVVHDF-PEX
Performer	Rand	4****	5–500	0–500	20 L	Y	Y	Pre Post	4	Y Y	1	IHD-IHFD-IHF, PEX- PAP - SCUF - CVVH - CVVHD-CVVHFD- CVVHFD
Prisma	Gambro	4	0–180	0–40	5 L	Blood warmer	Y	Pre Post Pre-Post	4	no Y	3	SCUF - CVVH - CVVHDCVVHFD - CVVHDF - PEX
Multifiltrate	FMC	4	0–500	0–70	24 L	Y in-line	Y	Pre Post Pre-Post	4	no Y	4	SCUF - CVVH — HV-HF CVVHD CVVHFD - CVVHDF —PEX
Prismaflex	Gambro	5	0–450	0–133	15 L	Y in-line	Y	Pre Post Pre-BP	5	no Y	4	SCUF - CVVH — HV-HF CVVHD CVVHFD - CVVHDF —PEX

* 2 pumps + 2 intelligent clamps;

** the 3 pumps for dialysate and fluid replacement are positioned inside the hydraulic circuit of the monitor

*** every pump runs two tubing segments;

**** the machine is equipped with thermal sensors.

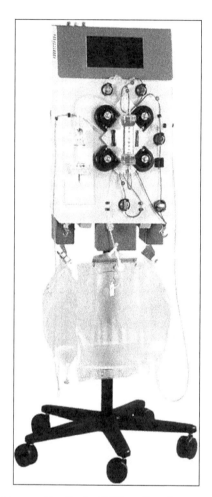

Figure 30.3 The Prisma machine. The first CRRT specific equipment ever developed.

are now equipped with a computer port that allows complete data extraction and the possibility of exporting data to populate a spreadsheet or database. Some machines are even equipped with built-in printers with automatic printing of the data at the end of the session. The transportability of the machine is an important aspect to be considered because these treatments may be performed in different sites of the same hospital or even outside, especially in peripheral units or disaster areas. The structure of the machines includes, in most of the cases, a practical trolley that effects easy movement of the equipment.

Technical Characteristics of Common CRRT Machines

The Prisma

The Prisma machine (Gambro-Sweden) is the first integrated equipment designed specifically for CRRT. It features a preassembled cartridge that includes lines and the filter. Tubing loading is automatic, as is the priming procedure. The presence of four pumps and three independent scales allows performance of all CRRT treatments. Blood flows can vary from 0 to 180 mL/min; dialysate flow ranges between 0 mL/min and 40 mL/min.

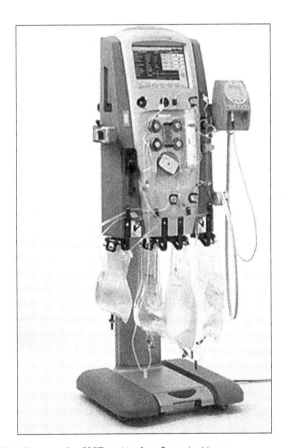

Figure 30.4 The prismaflex CRRT machine from Baxter healthcare.

The fluid handling capacity is 5 L. Pre-, post- and simultaneous pre-/post modes are available (Figure 30.3).

The Prismaflex Machine

The Prismaflex machine (Gambro-Sweden) presents features designed specifically to perform therapies with high fluid volume exchange, currently supposedly effective in acute renal failure, sepsis, and MODS. The machine features five pumps (blood, dialysate, preblood pump [PBP] replacement solution, postblood pump replacement solution, and effluent),four scales (effluent, dialysate and two for replacement solutions), and a disposable set

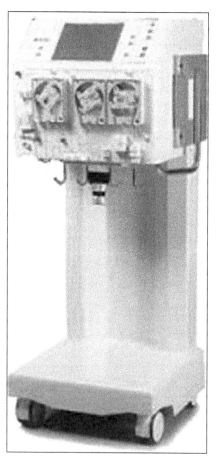

Figure 30.5 The Diapact machine from B. Braun.

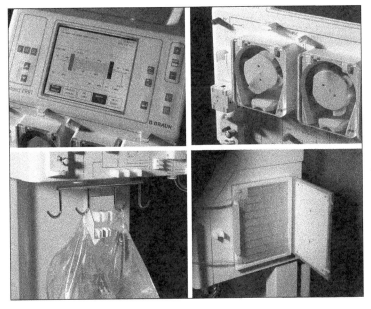

Figure 30.6 Details of the Diapact machine: The screen with pressure display, the pumps, the fluid bags and the dialysate warmer.

with preconnected high-flow filters and fluid circuitry. The machine allows the performance of a complete spectrum of therapies: slow, continuous ultrafiltration; CVVH; CVVHD; CVVHDF; therapeutic plasma exchange/PEx; and hemoperfusion. Three different preconnected kits with different surface-area filters for adult treatments are available—the M100 (the same as the Prisma set with AN69 membrane), the HF 1000, and the HF 1400 (Figure 30.4)—which have a larger surface (0.60, 1.00, and 1.40 m², respectively) and are especially useful in high-volume therapies. The last two also have different membranes (polyarylethersulfone). Contrary to the previous configuration in the classic Prisma machine, in the Primaflex the blood inlet is at the bottom of the filter, facilitating the priming procedure and elimination of air bubbles from the blood compartment. The innovative technical solution of two pinch valves provides the ability of varying the ratio between pre- and postdilution with different simultaneous infusion rates. This ratio can also be changed during therapy. Pre- or postdilution mode can also be selected for the CVVHDF modality. A heparin syringe pump was designed to accommodate different types and sizes of syringes. Another innovative feature is now present in the Prismaflex machine: the fifth pump. This pump delivers PBP fluid infusion and it makes possible to use citrate for circuit anticoagulation. This feature, in fact,

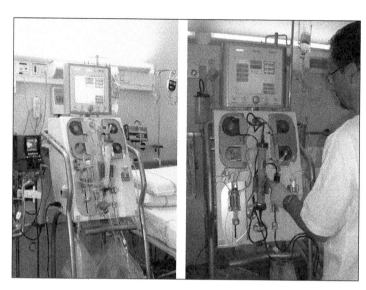

Figure 30.7 The Acquarius/Accura machine (Nikkiso).

allows citrate infusion just after the connection between the arterial access and the blood line.

The blood pump is bigger than in the earlier version and it allows blood flows within a range of 10–450 mL/min (depending on the filter in use). Fluid flow rate allows a maximum fluid handling of 8000 mL/h, both in hemofiltration and in hemodiafiltration. If PBP replacement solution is used, fluxes can be increased further. In this case, the blood pump is able to adjust its rotational speed automatically to maintain the prescribed blood flow, which otherwise would be relatively decreased by the scaling down factor induced by PBP infusion. Total effluent delivery ranges from 0 to 10,000 mL/h, allowing a maximum ultrafiltration of 2000 mL/h combined with the maximum dialysate/replacement flow rate. All these schemes are clearly designed to meet the issue of high-volume hemofiltration. Prismaflex software controls fluid flows by an accurate pump–scales feedback; 30 g/h is the accepted error for each pump and an alarm warns the operator if this limit is exceeded. The accuracy warranty is ensured further by an end-of-treatment setup, in case of scale damage or need for calibration. When the therapy is interrupted by a pressure alarm, it restarts automatically if the pressure level normalizes within few seconds (i.e., during coughs or inadvertent line kinking resulting from patients movement). Scales have become four parallel, sliding "drawers" positioned below the monitor, which can be shifted out and allow easy and back-safe collection of fluid bags. One of the most frequent concerns, the air removal chamber clots, has been challenged by an

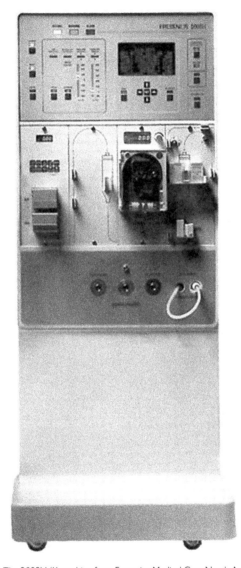

Figure 30.8 The 2008H/K machine from Fresenius Medical Care North America.

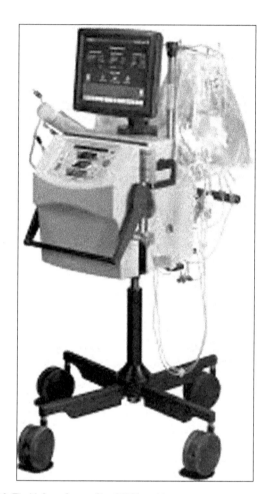

Figure 30.9 The NxStage System One (NSO) machine.

innovative design; the chamber is connected by a line to a pressure sensor that is able to adjust chamber blood levels via a pump. A reversed cone inside the chamber makes the blood run into the return line with a whirling movement, which reduces stagnant flows. Furthermore, when replacement solution is reinfused postfilter, it is poured directly on top of this cone to create a fluid layer between air and blood.

Sets are completed with 9-L effluent collection bags, which makes much more feasible the application of high-volume therapies without generating an excessive workload for ICU nurses. The colored monitor displays pressures and flows on the first screen, and complete graphs and events are listed in history pages. A PCMCIA card allows downloading of the data to laptop computers. Among the new features, filters with a modified and treated surface (ST 60, ST 100, ST 150) are today available with various surface area in different kits.

The Diapact CRRT

The Diapact machine (B.Braun, Melsungen) is derived from a series of prototypes called *emergency case units* or *ECUs*. The system has three pumps

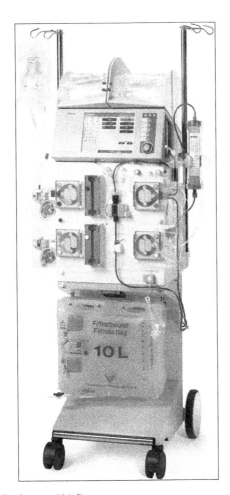

Figure 30.10 The Fresenius Multifiltrate.

with a wide range of blood flow (10–500 mL/min) and dialysate flow (5–400 mL/min) (Figures 30.5 and 30.6). Fluid handling and ultrafiltration control is gravimetric with one scale. Dialysate is warmed and the heparin pump is included. Reinfusion can be performed in either pre- or postdilution mode during hemofiltration. The machine is particularly suited for continuous high-flux hemodialysis, with the possibility of operating either in single-pass or recirculation mode.

The Acquarius/Accura

The Acquarius/Accura machine (Edwards Life Sciences) is a modern machine for CRRT (Figure 30.7). The system includes four pumps and two scales with the option of performing all CRRT treatments. Blood flow can be varied from 0 to 450 mL/min, and the dialysate flow rate ranges from 0 to 165 mL/min. The system includes a preassembled tubing set and a wide color screen with a user-friendly interface. The priming procedure is automatic. A fluid heater and heparin pump are included in the machine. Two independent scales allow for accurate and continuous fluid balancing whereas four pressure sensors help monitor extracorporeal circuit function. Pre-, post-, and simultaneous pre-/postdilution modes are available. Remarkable flexibility and versatility characterize this machine.

The 2008H/K

The 2008H/K machine (Fresenius Medical Care, Walnut Creek) is basically a standard intermittent hemodialysis machine that has been adapted to CRRT, and mostly sustained low-efficiency diafiltration, by modifying the software and the operational parameters (Figure 30.8). The machine is equipped with a blood pump plus three pumps for dialysate, which are internal. Blood flow can vary from 0 to 500 mL/min whereas the dialysate flow in CRRT mode can be set at three fixed values of 100, 200, and 300 mL/min. Dialysate is warmed and the heparin pump is built in. The system does not include a replacement pump, therefore hemofiltration modalities cannot be performed. The ultrafiltration control is open volumetric.

The NxStage System One

The NxStage System One (NSO) was developed to simplify CRRT treatments using new approaches in system design and technology (Figure 30.9). The key technological differentiator of the NSO is its use of a disposable cartridge containing all the blood and fluid pathways, including a volumetric fluid management system. This volumetric system balances fresh replacement fluid or dialysate with effluent coming from the dialyzer and removes excess fluid (net ultrafiltration) from the patient. The system allows the user to hang up to 29 L of replacement fluid or dialysate at one time and to connect the effluent directly to a drain with an air break. This approach minimizes the number of bag changes for the user to one or two per day, depending on the treatment prescription, and eliminates the need

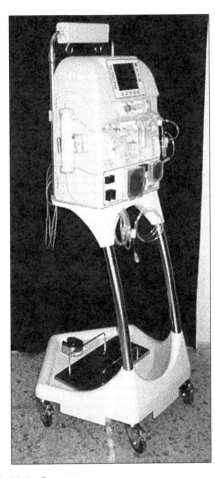

Figure 30.11 The Medica Equasmart.

to use (and empty) waste collection bags. The NSO does not use scales and is not subject to alarms resulting from bumping, moving, or swinging bags. The disposable cartridge loads into the NSO by opening the slide-out front door, placing the cartridge into the opening, and closing the door. All sensors, pumps, and actuators are loaded in this single step. After the user connects a 1-L saline prime bag to the cartridge and presses one button, the NSO primes the cartridge and verifies all hardware/disposable interfaces. This prime and testing process is accomplished without intervention from the user. The NSO can deliver intermittent or continuous therapies for continuous venovenous

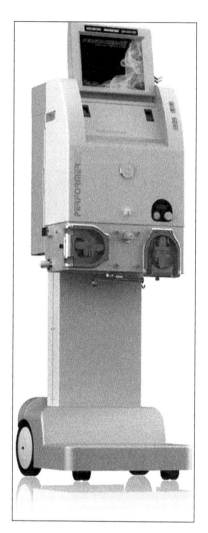

Figure 30.12 The RAND MOST Performer Machine.

hemofiltration CVVHF pre- or postdilution; CVVHD; slow, continuous ultra-filtration; and therapeutic plasma exchange therapies. However, the system does not perform CVVHDF. The blood pump speed range is 10 to 600 mL/min. The replacement fluid or dialysate rate is 0 to 12 L/h. The net ultrafiltration rate is 0 to 2.4 L/h. To reduce the risk of clotting, the cartridge does not

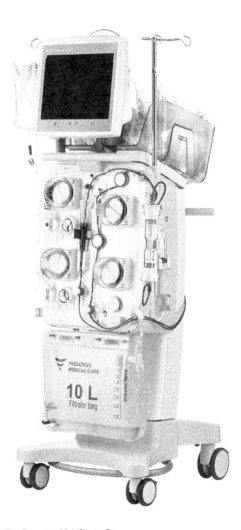

Figure 30.13 The Fresenius Multifiltrate Pro.

have air–blood interfaces. Pressure sensing on the cartridge is done through airless pods or directly in the tubing/flow paths. Air sensors are located on the arterial, replacement, and venous lines. Blood leak detection is located in the effluent line. Information generated by the NSO can also be ported to electronic medical record systems.

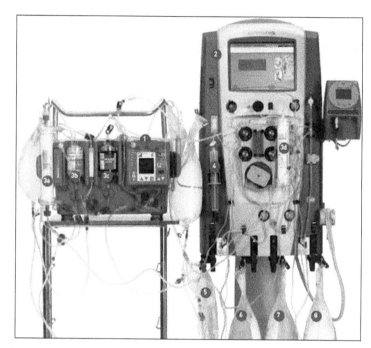

Figure 30.14 The Primaflex Mars combination for liver support.

The Fresenius Multifiltrate

This machine (Figure 30.10) has allowed to carry over treatments with large amount of fluid exchange such as high volume hemofiltration (HVHF) and Pulse high volume hemofiltration (PHVHF). The machine has been equipped quite early with a citrate anticoagulation feature allowing also to use any filter without captive preassembled disposable. The machine also features a step-by-step software with the possibility to follow the different phases of the treatment with a clear and well designed screen. The machine is only available in Europe.

The Medica Equasmart

Another machine designed to perform any CRRT treatment is the Medica Equasmart (Figure 30.11). This machine was one of the first equipped with a built in printer to summarize the data of the treatment and a built-it warmer. The machine can be used with any type of filter.

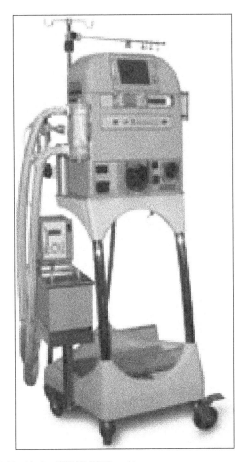

Figure 30.15 The Medica DECAP-CRRT machine.

Current and Future Technology

The evolution of CRRT has brought the concept of MOST: Multiple Organ Support Therapy. With this concept, the CRRT machine becomes a "platform" for extracorporeal therapies. Today, a fourth generation of machines for CRRT has been created, and further developments are planned for the years to come. The original simple machinery with blood pump and ultrafiltration/replacement pumps has been replaced by new, complex hardware in which five or six pumps are present, allowing one to perform almost any type of extracorporeal

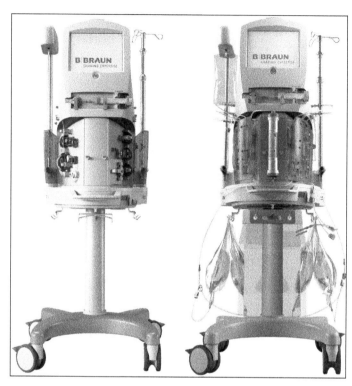

Figure 30.16 The B.Braun OMNI machine.

therapy designed for organ support. Anticoagulation regimes such as citrate may rely on dedicated hardware components. A large display is almost the rule for a more user-friendly interface. A large volume of fluid handling is ensured by precision scales, and blood or dialysate can be warmed for better comfort for the patient. New-generation machines have allowed to support different organ function with specific modalities. A new generation of machines is appearing on the scene. Some of them have not reached their full clinical application yet; nevertheless, they represent the future of this field. In addition to the safety of the therapy application being essential, the safeguarding of a smooth treatment performance and efficient use of resources have become significantly more important.

One example is the RAND MOST Performer (Figure 30.12) that not only makes possible to perform different therapies to support Heart, Liver, Kidney and Lung, but also has made possible the performance of locoregional pharmacological or thermal therapies.

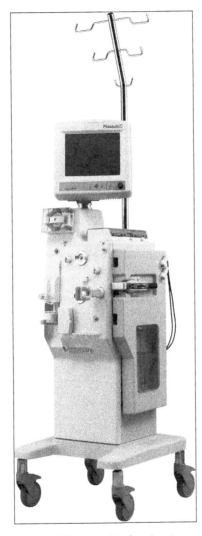

Figure 30.17 The Asahi medical Plasauto machine for apheresis.

Fresenius Medical Care has launched the Multifiltrate Pro (Figure 30.13), which is designed and engineered to fit the requirement of long-lasting, easy-to-use smooth CRRT therapy with a limited end user workload. In particular, fully integrated citrate anticoagulation and superflux membranes enable an effective treatment of acute kidney injury as well as multiple-organ failure.

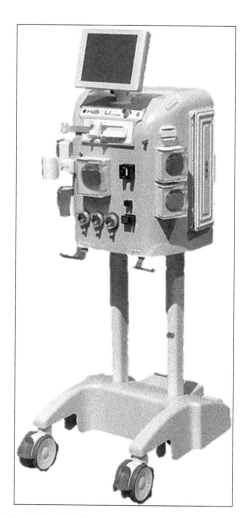

Figure 30.18 The Asahi medical Kibou machine for CRRT.

Baxter will launch the Prismax, which is an evolution of the Prismaflex. In the meantime the Prismaflex machine has been combined with the MARS circuit for the treatment of liver failure (Figure 30.14) or with a small oxygenator to remove CO2 and support the lungs in case of hypercapnia, allowing ultraprotective mechanical ventilation. Medica has also developed a machine capable to perform extracorporal CO2 removal in combination with CRRT

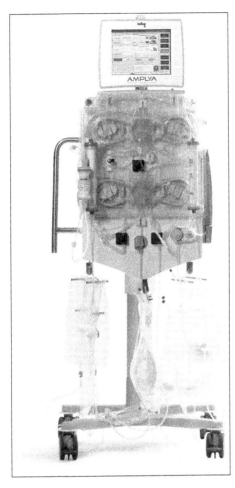

Figure 30.19 The Amplya Machine for CRRT and CPFA.

(Figure 30.15). B.Braun has launched a new CRRT machine called OMNI (Figure 30.16) with full capability for administering all extracorporeal therapies. This machine represents a real step forward in comparison with the previous Diapact machine. ASAHI has recently proposed the Plasauto system (Figure 30.17) and this machine is basically utilized for therapeutic apheresis. The company however has entered the field of CRRT with the newly designed Kibou CRRT machine (Figure 30.18). Bellco has developed a system for

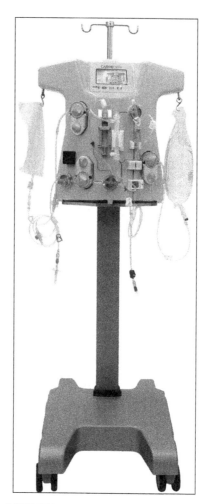

Figure 30.20 The CARPEDIEM machine for CRRT in neonates.

Coupled Plasma Filtration Adsorption (CPFA) application and has launched a new integrated machine called Amplya (Figure 30.19). The same company has made a great deal of effort to develop, in conjunction with the International Renal Research Institute of Vicenza, a specifically designed machine for neonates called Carpediem (Figure 30.20). This machine is unique being specifically designed for neonates and infants enabling CRRT in babies less than 3 Kg. Estor, in conjunction with Toray, has developed a machine called

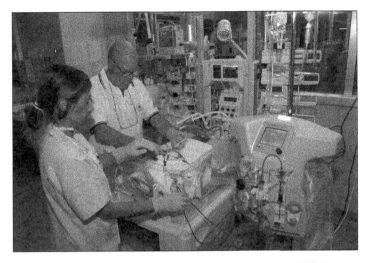

Figure 30.21 The first neonate in the world treated with the miniaturized CARPEDIEM Machine.

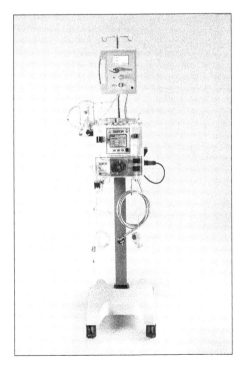

Figure 30.22 The Estorflow machine for HP and ECCO2R.

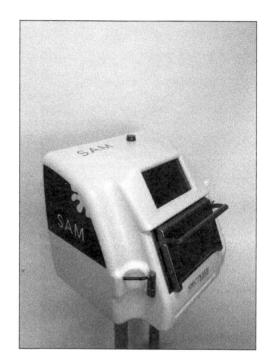

Figure 30.23 The Spectral SAM machine.

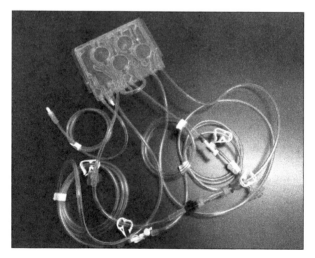

Figure 30.24 The disposable cassette with blood and dialysate circuit and pump segments.

Estorflow which is capable of performing Polymyxin-B hemoperfusion and extracorporeal CO_2 removal (Figure 30.22). Although other machines have been recently adapted to remove CO_2 through small oxygenators placed in series with a CRRT circuit or as a stand-alone therapy, this machine is the only one equipped with online measurement of CO_2 removal. Spectral company in Canada has recently presented the Spectral Apheresis Machine (SAM), a new, advanced extracorporeal treatment platform designed to perform various CRRT and sustained low-efficiency hemodiafiltration techniques, as well as other extracorporeal therapies, such as direct hemoperfusion and CO_2 removal (Figure 30.23). The system uses a synchronized piston pump system run by four internal cam shafts that also run the pump clamps. This piston-driven system has demonstrated less hemolysis during preliminary testing versus a traditional occlusive rotary pump. The compact nature of the cam-driven system allows for the use of a compact, solid disposable cassette that can be inserted into the machine in one simple step (Figure 30.24). When this cassette is installed, the pressure monitoring system, pumps, clamps, chambers, and blood leak and air detectors are all connected automatically in parallel. The simplicity of loading the cassette makes the installation of the tubing set nearly effortless, as well as reduces machine setup time drastically. The compact nature of the system also means that SAM is one of the smallest extracorporeal platforms available, without lacking any key features.

SAM is supplied with several different disposables for various treatments, including a cassette that is less restrictive than those provided for other CRRT machines. This open system allows SAM to be more flexible than other CRRT machines, permitting a very wide variety of treatment applications. SAM is currently under final development by Spectral Medical Inc., and its planned launch to the European and North American market is by the end of 2016.

In conclusion, all these new platforms will likely make CRRT safer and simpler, and allow clinicians to perform therapy more efficiently and safely.

An important evolution in CRRT technology is taking place in this moment with development and placement on the market of brand new machines for CRRT but beyond them, new models of connectivity, electronics and human interface are under evaluation. The years to come will therefore see a further evolution of this therapy or group of therapies for a better care of our patients.

Key References

Bellomo R, Baldwin I, Cole L, Ronco C. Preliminary experience with high volume hemofiltration in human septic shock. *Kidney Int.* 1998;53(suppl 66):S182–S185.

Bellomo R, Ronco C. Continuous versus intermittent renal replacement therapy in the intensive care unit. *Kidney Int.* 1998;53(suppl 66):S125–S128.

Clark WR, Ronco C. Renal replacement therapy in acute renal failure: solute removal mechanism and dose quantification. *Kidney Int.* 1998;53(suppl 66):S133–S137.

Geronemus R, Schneider N. Continuous arterio-venous hemodialysis: a new modality for treatment of acute renal failure. *Trans ASAIO.* 1984;30:610–613.

Kramer P, Wigger W, Rieger J, Matthaei D, Scheler F. Arteriovenous hemofiltration: a new and simple method for treatment of over hydrated patients resistant to diuretics. *Klin Wocherr-Scrift.* 1997;55:1121–1122.

Rahmati S, Ronco F, Spittle M, et al. Validation of the blood temperature monitor for extracorporeal thermal energy balance during in vitro continuous hemodialysis. *Blood Purif.* 2001;19: 245–250.

Ronco C. Arterio-venous hemodiafiltration (AVHDF): a possible way to increase urea removal during CAVH. *Int J of Artif Organs.* 1985;8:61–62.

Ronco C. Continuous renal replacement therapies for the treatment of acute renal failure in intensive care patients. *Clin Nephrol.* 1993;4:187–198.

Ronco C. Continuous renal replacement therapies in the treatment of acute renal failure in intensive care patients. Part 1: theoretical aspects and techniques. *Nephrol Dial Transplant.* 1994;9(suppl 4):191–200.

Ronco C, Bellomo R. Complications with continuous renal replacement therapies. *Am J Kidney Dis.* 1996;28(5 suppl 3):100–104.

Ronco C, Bellomo R. Continuous renal replacement therapy: evolution in technology and current nomenclature. *Kidney Int.* 1998;53(suppl 66):S160–S164.

Ronco C, Bellomo R. *Critical Care Nephrology.* Dordrecht, Netherlands: Kluwer Academic Publishers; 1998.

Ronco C, Bellomo R, Homel P, et al. Effects of different doses in continuous veno-venous haemofiltration on outcomes of acute renal failure: a prospective randomised trial. *Lancet.* 2000;356:26–30.

Ronco C, Brendolan A, Bellomo R. Current technology for continuous renal replacement therapies. In: Ronco C, Bellomo R, eds. *Critical Care Nephrology.* Dordrecht: Kluwer Academic Publishers; 1998:1269–1308.

Ronco C, Brendolan A, Bellomo R. On-line monitoring in continuous renal replacement therapies. *Kidney Int.* 1999;56(suppl 72):S8–S14.

Ronco C, Burchardi H. Management of acute renal failure in the critically ill patient. In: Pinsky MR, Dhaunaut JFA, eds. *Pathophysiobiologic Foundations of Critical Care.* Baltimore: Williams and Wilkins; 1993:630–676.

Ronco C, Ghezzi P, Bellomo R. New perspective in the treatment of acute renal failure. *Blood Purif.* 1999;17:166–172.

Ronco C, Garzotto F, Brendolan A, et al. Continuous renal replacement therapy in neonates and small infants: development and first-in-human use of a miniatursed machine (CARPEDIEM). Lancet. 2014;383(9931):1807–1813.

Tetta C, Bellomo R, Brendolan A, et al. Use of adsorptive mechanisms in continuous renal replacement therapies in the critically ill. *Kidney Int.* 1999;56(S72):S15–S19.

Tetta C, Cavaillon JM, Schulze M, et al. Removal of cytokines and activated complement components in an experimental model of continuous plasma filtration coupled with sorbent adsorption. *Nephrol Dial Transplant.* 1998;13:1458–1464.

Tetta C, Mariano F, Ronco C, Bellomo R. Removal and generation of inflammatory mediators during continuous renal replacement therapies. In: Ronco C, Bellomo R, eds. *Critical Care Nephrology.* Kluwer Academic Publishers; 1998:1239–1248.

Chapter 31

Quality Improvement for Continuous Renal Replacement Therapies

Ian Baldwin and Rinaldo Bellomo

There are different clinical parameters that can reflect the successful use of continuous renal replacement therapy (CRRT) and the achievement of relevant therapeutic goals. The major goals of CRRT include desired toxic solute clearance, acid–base homeostasis, electrolyte balance, appropriate fluid removal and balance, and temperature control. These goals should, ideally, be achieved in a timely and cost-effective manner. Establishing and maintaining a unit CRRT database is useful to gauge success, compare unit performance with that of others, and enable review or change over time to detect potentially useful trends in performance. This quality improvement process is useful in respect to the changing clinical context, personnel changes and training requirements, new devices and CRRT machines, access devices, and technical variations in the prescription for anticoagulation and fluid balance.

Data collection can be done in the form of a specific "snapshot" assessment over a short period (e.g., 1 month) or done continuously. Common useful quality measures are listed here and summarized in Table 31.1. Here, we discuss some important aspects of quality improvement:

- *Daily review* of patient biochemistry and fluid balance for adequate volume control is vital. This would appear to be an obvious quality activity. However, a bedside review is useful, particularly when prescribing physicians and nurses change frequently for the same patient over many days. Fluid balance needs to be assessed to determine whether inputs exceed fluid loss. Fluid removed by the treatment does not necessarily mean a neutral or negative patient balance has been achieved. This is an important process to clarify in bedside discussions and treatment prescriptions to ensure goals are being achieved. Adequate written and formal documentation of fluid management goals and fluid balance is mandatory.
- *Number of patients treated*, duration of each treatment, and days of treatment for each patient are important, necessary data. Some ICU database schedules capture these data already. However, a review of these data is useful for a team providing CRRT. Individual treatment data can be

Table 31.1 Quality Indicators Associated with Renal Replacement Therapy

Quality Assurance Item	Clinical Comment
Daily review	Solutes, urea, and creatinine should be declining or stable each day. Fluid loss is usually required and should be achieved each day, considering all fluid inputs and losses, not those of the machine alone. An accurate patient weight is useful.
Number of patients treated	This piece of information is useful in staff level justification, budgeting, and notation of patterns of prescribing and number of machines in use.
Time without treatment	Time without treatment can reflect differences over 24-hour periods, staffing changes, training, and medical review. It may also reflect inadequate dosing and undertreatment, if excessive.
Errors, adverse events	Frequent mistakes reflect a need to change policy or add more training and resource development. For example, fluid balance mistakes may suggest misunderstanding of orders and how clinicians interpret fluid loss. Is this machine loss or patient net loss?
Access catheters used	How many access catheters are being used? Are they being replaced frequently? Such data suggest a need to change methods, use a new design, and/or review and amend maintenance and care routines, such as management of the device when not used, how the dressing, is placed and secured.
Cost of consumables	It useful to have up-to-date knowledge of consumables costs and then determine the average cost for each patient, The total cost of all consumables and number of patients treated annually indicates the cost per patient.
No and attendees at education sessions	Review how many education sessions are being provided that focus on CRRT, and the number or percent of staff attending. Focus on clinicians understanding the CRRT circuit.

CRRT, continuous renal replacement therapy.

maintained on bedside charts/computers and is very helpful in monitoring success and failure in a patient. Sequential, progressive charting of a treatment, with each new treatment starting again at hour 1, achieves this and provides a quick assessment for time on treatment or filter life. A common filter life using CRRT across all patients in the ICU is a median of 20 consecutive hours. The mean value is often skewed by outlying data: one very long or short treatment.

• *The time without treatment* or "off time" in each patient ICU stay. The time when renal replacement therapy is not occurring, or downtime, is a useful measure of efficiency because solute levels will rise with increasing downtime. There are many reasons for extended periods without CRRT being applied, despite a continuous prescription. However, these data can reflect inefficient practices, lack of nursing staff and skill, delayed medical review, the frequent need for out-of-ICU diagnostics, and bad policies. Such data are often not reported. However, publications indicate that a downtime of approximately \5 hours for each 24 hours may be common.

- *Errors, adverse events* and mistakes, specific alarm events, and machine repairs are relatively common. Although many mistakes and malfunctions are not reported, or lack surrounding context data, these data provide useful feedback to the CRRT team. Such data must be managed with sensitivity and be used to improve CRRT in a constructive manner, avoiding individuals being targeted. Frequent identical events reflect a need to change and modify policy. Where many CRRT machines exist, naming or numbering each machine makes tracking of machines and repairs or failures easier.

- *Access catheters used* and microbiology associated with clinical use. Access devices can be overlooked as separate from therapy. The number used and type and site of insertion provide useful data. A database with information on such devices, site of insertion, time of insertion, date of insertion, person who inserted the device, and complications related to insertion or subsequent catheter colonization, infection, or vessel thrombosis are very useful in monitoring the safety and quality of catheter management.

Table 31.2 Potential CRRT Problems and Responses

Problem	Response
Frequent filter clotting in unit	Review nurse education. Review anticoagulation policies. Review site and choice of vascular access catheter.
Frequent filter clotting in individual patients	Review circumstances around episode. Check resistance of outflow/inflow in access catheter. Check choice of vascular access site. Review patient position and movement. Review anticoagulation approach.
Long downtime	Review nurse training. Emphasize need to prime circuit quickly. See previous responses to frequent filter clotting.
Errors in fluid balance	Optimize physician and nurse education. Chart fluid balance accurately and ensure clarity of medical prescription of desired fluid balance.
Patient on vasopressor therapy and hypotension	Initiate CRRT slowly. Begin with slow blood flow (20–30 mL/min) for more than 5 minutes until the circuit is filled with blood and blood is returning to the patient. Increase the blood pump flow slowly to the desired rate by 20–50-mL/min increments. Initiate therapy only after the blood flow is at the desired level. If necessary, increase vasopressor drug therapy by 10% to 20% before the start of CRRT or administer a small fluid bolus . This fuid can be removed after therapy has been established.
Unexplained fever or leukocytosis	Examine vascular access site. Consider removal of catheter (guidewire exchange preferred as initial step).
Swollen limb distal to catheter	Consider deep venous thrombosis. Perform ultrasound. If a large clot is present, initiate anticoagulation. Do not remove the catheter immediately because this can trigger a lethal embolism.

CRRT, continuous renal replacement therapy.

- *Cost of consumables*—circuits and any device or component used for the CRRT circuit. This information provides feedback for managers and helps with decision making on purchasing and supply contracts.

Table 31.2 lists potential CRRT problems and appropriate responses.

Summary

Collection and review of patient daily biochemistry, filter life, and time without treatment all provide useful measures of CRRT quality. Biochemistry should reflect solute reduction, filter life should be approximately 20 hours, and time without treatment should be minimal. Reviewing adverse events, machine repairs, and simple mistakes and errors is necessary to prevent serious harm during CRRT. Such information helps guide effective education and policy development. Cost data can be a measure of success; increasing costs are associated with inefficient treatments, access catheter malfunction, and poor filter life. The safety and quality of CRRT are highly dependent on the collection of quality improvement data. If this is not done, the quality and safety of CRRT are seriously undermined, and patients are exposed to a risk of major complications.

Key References

Baldwin I. Factors affecting circuit patency and filter life. *Contrib Nephrol.* 2007;156:178–184.

Baldwin I, Bellomo R. Relationship between blood flow, access catheter and circuit failure during CRRT: a practical review. *Contrib Nephrol.* 2004;144:203–213.

Baldwin I, Tan HK, Bridge N, Bellomo R. Possible strategies to prolong circuit life during hemofiltration: three controlled studies. *Renal Fail.* 2002;24(6):839–848.

Boyle M, Baldwin I. Understanding the continuous renal replacement therapy circuit for acute renal failure support: a quality issue in the intensive care unit. *AACN Adv Crit Care.* 2010;21(4):365–375.

Lipcsey M, Chua HR, Schneider AG, Robbins R, Bellomo R. Clinically manifest complications of femoral vein catheterization for continuous renal replacement therapy. *J Crit Care.* 2043;29:18–23.

Ronco C, Ricci Z, Bellomo R, Baldwin I, Kellum J. Management of fluid balance in CRRT: a technical approach. *Int J Artif Organs.* 2005;28(8):765–776.

Uchino S, Fealy N, Baldwin I, Morimatsu H, Bellomo R. Pre-dilution vs. post-dilution during continuous veno-venous hemofiltration: impact on filter life and azotemic control. *Nephron Clin Pract.* 2003;94(4):c94–c98.

Chapter 32

Educational Resources

Ian Baldwin and Kimberly Whiteman

Continuous renal replacement therapy (CRRT) requires a significant commitment to ongoing education and training. Machines for CRRT are automated for the priming and preparation sequence; however, they can be challenging for new learners to master and operate safely. Fluid balance and anticoagulation regimens can be a source of mistakes without adequate education. It is also important to recognize that manufacturers' operating manuals for machines are not always suitably prepared for the clinical environment, and idiosyncrasies of clinical patient care when using a machine need to be developed and taught locally.

The application of theoretical frameworks to psychomotor clinical skills for CRRT is a challenge for the nursing instructor and is best achieved using a variety of approaches. The use of multiple teaching strategies recognizes that people learn in different ways and may need different experiences to gain knowledge and clinical skills. Instructional methods can include video or DVD review; system simulation exercises; circuit setup using suitable abstract models, such as drawing board exercises or computer diagrams; computerized instruction; priming practice with nonsterile circuits on machines when not in use; bedside instruction; and, last, real-life patient care experiences with and without supervision. Educational needs can be divided into introductory competency development and ongoing continuing education.

Introductory Education: Theory and Practical Training

Theory must accompany practical training. Nurses caring for patients on CRRT need to know the science behind treatments and how to operate the equipment safely. In addition, education about fluid balance and anticoagulation regimes helps to eliminate errors. Education delivery may vary depending on the setting, but the content that needs to be learned remains constant. A method of delivery for small groups of 8 to 12 nurses is a 1-day seminar, with theory in the morning and practical machine activities in the afternoon (Figure 32.1). The core content suggested here can be adapted to any learning environment or time frame.

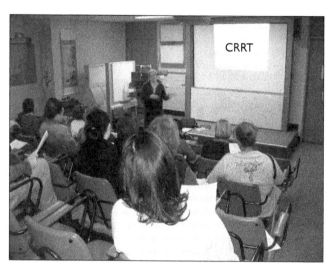

Figure 32.1 A continuous renal replacement therapy (CRRT) classroom for theory using a standard lecture set.

Theory can be taught as a lecture set with course handout notes and current journal references. Suggested lectures include the following content:

- Acute kidney injury and critical illness
  - Begin the course with a review of acute kidney injury and historical treatments, such as hemodialysis and peritoneal dialysis. Review that standard safety measures with central lines, such as radiographic confirmation of line placement, should be completed before treatment initiation. Include and emphasize that treatments should be initiated as soon as possible after the confirmation of line placement. Emphasize the need for immediate treatment of patients with severe electrolyte imbalances and not to wait for initiation of CRRT. For example, patients with high potassium levels should be treated with standard regimes such as insulin and glucose or sodium polystyrene sulfonate (Kayexylate) until CRRT can be started.
- Theory of solvent and solute removal
  - Describe the principles of ultrafiltration, diffusion, and convection. Discuss clearance of fluid and small molecules as the goal of treatment. Review commonly prescribed drugs and how blood levels can be affected by CRRT.
- Treatments of CRRT: slow continuous ultrafiltration, continuous venovenous hemofiltration, continuous venovenous hemodialysis, continuous venovenous hemodiafiltration

- Use diagrams and drawings to discuss the construction of the filter with hollow fibers, and the blood and fluid flow for each of the four possible treatments.
- With regard to diffusive techniques, the filter is a hemodialyzer with hollow fibers inside. The blood flows through the center of the hollow fibers, and the dialysate flows around the hollow fibers. Commonly, blood and fluid flow in opposite directions, which is called *countercurrent flow*.
- The fluid flow path varies slightly depending on the treatment. It is important for class participants to understand that dialysate fluid is not intended to enter the bloodstream. Dialysate flows around the hollow fibers, diffusion occurs, and waste is pumped directly into the effluent bag or dialysate drain along with any additional fluid removed from the patient during treatment. Depending on the manufacturer and the type of treatment, replacement fluids might enter the bloodstream before the filter (predilution) or after the filter (postdilution) or both.
- The blood path for all CRRT modalities mandates blood is pulled or sucked from the patient with negative pressure, enters the filter through tubing that is color-coded red (access), exits the filter, and is returned or pushed to the patient under positive pressure in lines color-coded blue (return).
- Fluids and fluid balance
  - Review the dialysis principles and blood and fluid flow used in each of the four types of CRRT.
    1. Slow continuous ultrafiltration: ultrafiltration
    2. Continuous venovenous hemofiltration: convection and ultrafiltration
    3. Continuous venovenous hemodialysis: diffusion and ultrafiltration
    4. Continuous venovenous hemodiafiltration: diffusion and convection
  - Discuss the components of net fluid balance for any given period of time.
    - Net fluid balance = All fluids in − All fluids out
    - Generally, the goal for fluid balance is a negative number or zero
  - Nurses performing CRRT should be aware of the daily fluid balance goals set for the patient. Periodically, throughout each shift or as frequently as prescribed, check to see whether the fluid balance goals are being achieved.
  - Emphasize that fluid and solute removal is calculated on the delivery of a continuous treatment. Prolonged, unplanned lapses in treatment should be avoided; when they occur, they may contribute to a positive fluid balance.
  - Review examples of clinical situations in which blood products or new orders for large volumes of antibiotics affect the net negative balance, along with how to mitigate the fluid gain.

- Review any site-specific protocols for achieving net negative goals. Protocols might include a standing order to call the physician if the net negative fluid balance goals are not met, or a protocol to increase fluid removal rates with blood transfusions or other large volumes of fluid, such as newly prescribed antibiotics.
- Manufacturers vary in regard to what fluids are calculated automatically into the machine fluid balance and what fluids need to be added separately into the intake and output. This information is important for calculating the intake and output.
- Anticoagulation protocol and potential complications
  - Discuss the reason for anticoagulation and review any site-specific protocols for administration and monitoring.
  - If citrate is used as an anticoagulant, review the calcium replacement protocol, ionized calcium monitoring, and signs and symptoms of hypocalcemia and hypercalcemia.
  - If heparin is used, review dosing, protamine reversal protocols, prothrombin time, and international normalization ratio normal values.
- Complications of CRRT
  - Discuss possible complications related to CRRT and how to prevent and treat them. Complications include hypotension, electrolyte imbalance, hypothermia, bleeding, blood leak, and infection.
  - Air embolism is a complication associated with the use of any extracorporeal circuit, and procedures for removing air should be taught and practiced in a simulated environment.
  - Special considerations for patients taking angiotensin-converting enzyme inhibitors may be required.

Other course materials may include the following:

- Excerpts from the manufacturer's operator manual can be reprinted with permission.
- References, lectures, and course material may also be placed on computers or intranet sites for reference.
- Hospital policy or protocol documents are an essential reference. As with many areas of intensive care machine management, a multidisciplinary consensus policy is useful as a "baseline" reference point for learners. Some new learners prefer a bulleted list of the descriptive steps and pictures in lieu of the procedure, which can be a long list when the rationale is added.
- Emergency procedures to be followed in case of cardiac arrest should be determined in an interprofessional forum and made available to clinicians. Consider including a scenario with a cardiac arrest or other emergency during the practical part of the course to provide experience with the psychomotor skills of managing an emergency with the CRRT equipment.

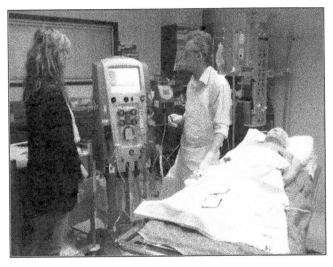

Figure 32.2 Continuous renal replacement therapy basic simulation with resuscitation doll and machine for demonstration of priming, patient connection, and common alarms.

Practical Experience

After the participants have gained an understanding of the theories behind treatment with CRRT, provide time to work with the machine to be used in clinical treatment (Figure 32.2).

The following components are suggestions for practical experience. For small classes, use a sequential model, with the whole class working through the skills. For larger classes, breakout sessions with multiple machines or stations and a final demonstration of synthesis of steps can help to save time and keep the participants engaged:

- Machines and extracorporeal circuit setup
  - In a controlled classroom environment, each nurse should be given the opportunity to set up and prime a machine. In larger classes, it may be necessary to work in pairs. Allow the nurses time to read on-screen directions and help screens.
- Care and maintenance of temporary dialysis catheter
  - Have the temporary dialysis catheters used in the clinical areas at your site available in class for participants to view and handle.
  - Discuss the anatomic placement of the temporary dialysis catheter. Double-lumen dialysis catheters (15–20 cm) placed in the right internal jugular vein have the most direct path to the right atria and tend to have

the best flow. Left internal jugular and femoral veins can also be used. Longer catheters (e.g., 24 cm) are used in the femoral vein only. This length of catheter is unsuitable for jugular or subclavian use. The subclavian site is generally used last to preserve its integrity in case a semipermanent dialysis catheter might need to be inserted later.

- Review the flow through the double-lumen dialysis catheter. One lumen is color-coded red and is sometimes referred to as the *access line*, because blood is pulled from the patient into the filter through this lumen. Blood is returned through the blue lumen or "return" that exits at the distal end of the catheter. When the catheter lumens are connected properly to the CRRT tubing lines, this design prevents recirculation of clean blood through the circuit.

- When CRRT is interrupted or discontinued, the temporary dialysis catheter is capped. End caps should not accommodate needle or intravenous entry. Often an anticoagulant, such as heparin, is instilled in the lumens. Lumens should be clearly labeled with the type and dose of anticoagulant. Consider placing a label or barrier over the end caps as a physical reminder to personnel that anticoagulant is present and needs to be withdrawn and discarded before use.

- Entrance into the temporary dialysis catheter and dressing changes should be performed using aseptic technique, and should follow hospital policies for dressings and sterile procedures.

- Two professional organizations provide evidence-based recommendations for care of temporary dialysis catheters and patients on CRRT and may be helpful in developing local policies and procedures:
  1. The Amercian Association of Critical Care Nurses: *AACN Procedure Manual for Critical Care*
  2. American Nephrology Nurses Association (ANNA): *Nephrology Nursing Process of Care: Apheresis and Therapeutic Plasma Exchange and Continuous Renal Replacement Therapy*

- To troubleshoot during nursing care of a patient on CRRT, use the acronym PACE:
  - *Patient*: Look at the patient first. Coughing, patient positioning, and movement can sometimes set off circuit alarms.
  - *Access*: Access refers to the temporary dialysis catheter. Check for a blood return and flow before starting treatment and for patency, kinks, or clamps when alarms occur. Consider teaching a standard access troubleshooting sequence, such as the following example:
    - Release kinks in the catheter
    - Reposition the patient
    - Reposition the catheter
    - Attempt to flush the catheter
  - *Circuit*: The circuit is the disposable filter and tubing. Clots or gas bubbles can cause alarms. Teach participants to remove air from lines using manufacturers' guidelines, inspect the filter for clots, and use the pressures

measured by the machine to determine where problems are located within the circuit. For example, highly negative access pressure may be indicative of access line kinking.

- *Equipment*: Equipment failure or power outages can cause a disruption in care. The machine should be plugged into the emergency power source to permit automatic switching to backup power in case of an outage. Procedures for equipment failure should be developed and reviewed in class.
- Alarm conditions
  - Common alarm conditions can be simulated easily in the classroom setting.
  - Suggested alarms that should be simulated in class include access (high negative pressure) and return line (high positive pressure) kinks, air in line, and alarms that require nursing intervention, such as fluid bag changing and fluid balance settings.
  - Nurses should be aware that repeated alarms should be investigated thoroughly. Consider a "three strikes" policy that requires nurses to seek help if they are unable to remedy an alarm on the third try (Figure 32.3).
- Termination of treatment
  - Review the sequence for termination of treatment. Consider combining this simulation with a scenario that includes flushing the temporary dialysis catheter, instilling anticoagulant, and labeling.
  - If desired, develop and practice a protocol for recirculation or temporary disconnection for off-unit interventions, such as in radiology or the operating room.
  - Discuss signs of a blood leak or rupture of the filter, including blood in the effluent. Instruct participants to discontinue treatment without returning the blood to the patient in cases of confirmed blood leaks.
- Documentation

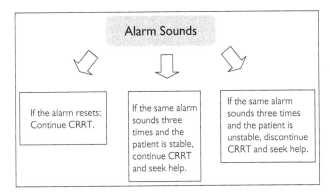

Alarm Sounds

| If the alarm resets: Continue CRRT. | If the same alarm sounds three times and the patient is stable, continue CRRT and seek help. | If the same alarm sounds three times and the patient is unstable, discontinue CRRT and seek help. |

Figure 32.3 Troubleshooting tree. CRRT, continuous renal replacement therapy.

- Teach participants to document the following according to local policy:
  - Patient and family education regarding the CRRT procedure
  - Condition of the catheter insertion site
  - Intake and output

Whenever possible, use actual bedside documentation tools in class. Use several hours of data for intake and output measurements, and check that all participants can complete the charting accurately.

Learning Environment

Offer a variety of practical approaches for learning. Develop methods for teaching CRRT that appeal to a variety of learning styles, including the following:

- Video- or computer-assisted instruction for review or individual learning
- Cue cards or quick reference charts that can be kept with the machine after class
- Troubleshooting tutorials or scenarios that include common alarm conditions and potential complications of treatment such as hypothermia, air embolism, and frequent filter clotting
- Case exemplars that include common errors in clinical practice such as fluid balance and anticoagulation errors
- Mentored real-life experience with CRRT in which expert nurses provide an extended time for practical learning of skills after class participation
- A competency checklist that includes critical skills: setup, on and off procedures for connecting to the temporary dialysis catheter, termination of treatment

This varied approach to learning can link the sequence of abstract discussion, simulation, and then real-life experience (Figure 32.4).

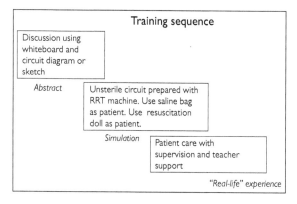

Figure 32.4 Suggested learning sequence useful in continuous renal replacement therapy education. RRT, renal replacement therapy.

Assessment of Learning

Quizzes, demonstrations of key skills by the participants, or other measurements of learning should be developed. Participation in a debriefing session after troubleshooting simulations or real-life experience can help with development of critical thinking skills. Encourage learners to describe their understanding of why alarms and problems occur, in addition to their suggested remedy to demonstrate their understanding. This activity is in contrast to simply correcting the problem each time.

Observation of clinical practice can be evaluated after the formal class day either by the instructor or by CRRT clinical experts on the units.

CRRT Champion

After initial training, bedside experts are necessary to sustain a program. A nurse instructor or experienced clinical nurse on staff is necessary to "champion" CRRT and link education and clinical implementation. The CRRT champion needs to be able to work with other disciplines within the organization and with the manufacturer to coordinate care of patients. Periodic updates to standards and policies need to be completed and disseminated. New research and techniques should be reviewed and considered for implementation into practice. A multidisciplinary team approach to care helps to ensure patients receive safe and effective care. The CRRT champion can serve as the coordinator of the team (Figure 32.5).

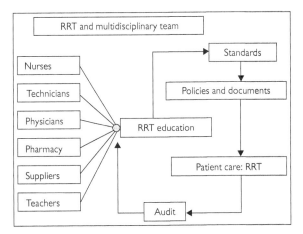

Figure 32.5 The continuous renal replacement therapy educator is central to others involved and is a "champion" for this specialized aspect of nursing in the intensive care unit. RRT, renal replacement therapy.

Box 32.1 Definitions: Key Terms Associated with RRT

abstract model an activity using some aspects of simulation to prepare for real events using concepts with readily available representative materials (e.g., use simple cut-out pictures of renal replacement therapy machines and components rather than the machine itself)

competency being able to perform a task or skill within a set time with no mistakes; able to recognize an error and fix it

education a process that provides instruction and information for analysis and knowledge development; responding to cognition

lecture a series of topics designed and presented in sequence; used when information is sensitive to logical flow in learning from simple to complex

real-life experience undertaking tasks and applying knowledge previously learned in a simulation or education process in a real, nonartificial situation

simulation an activity that copies real-life events for learners to develop knowledge without fear of mistakes and to seek feedback when they fail or lack competency

troubleshooting recognizing an error and applying remedies to correct the error with effect

Competency and Ongoing Education

Nurses will be exposed to patients on CRRT at varying levels, depending upon the medical practice and patient care needs. The CRRT educator or champion should plan for programs to ensure ongoing competence of staff on an as-needed or yearly basis. Topics for competency education should be selected based on institutional needs. Quality and risk management reports, as well as manufacturer changes to machine hardware and software, can be used to develop updates for clinical staff. Nurses who frequently perform CRRT may have different yearly competencies and learning needs than those who seldom perform the skills. Consider competencies based on theory, and skills needed for setting up, maintaining, and discontinuing treatment. Track questions asked of the nurse educator to determine common or frequently asked questions to consider for yearly education. Information from alarm or treatment history recorded in the machines or maintenance records may be used to determine frequent problems. Review of risk management or quality data, such as temporary dialysis catheter-associated infections, can also be used to plan competency education. New knowledge or advances in treatment should be reviewed when available, but at least yearly, with all staff caring for patients on CRRT.

Consider the development of an advanced CRRT user program or unit-based expert development program. This program could include more in-depth troubleshooting and current trends in practice taken from the literature. Advanced users could also be mentors or preceptors for nurses who have recently begun caring for patients on CRRT, providing for supervised real-life learning experience.

Summary

Skilled care of patients with CRRT in the intensive care unit is a specialized area of knowledge for nurses. As with mechanical ventilation and cardiac support devices, it takes time to learn the "language," make sense of the treatment prescription, and master the machines that are used to provide treatment. Theory, abstract learning, simulation, and live experience with supervision all facilitate learning and the development of clinical expertise. An experienced nurse champion who has been educated in the care of patients on CRRT is an effective way to achieve positive outcomes in a busy intensive care unit environment.

Key References

Baldwin I, Fealy N. Clinical nursing for the application of continuous renal replacement therapy in the intensive care unit. *Semin Dial.* 2009;22(2):189–193.

Cope G. The basic principles of continuous renal replacement therapy. *J Renal Nurs.* 2013;5(2):85–91.

Dennison HA. Creating a computer-assisted learning module for the non-expert nephrology nurse. *Nephrol Nurs J.* 2011;38(1):41–53.

Dirkes S. Acute kidney injury: not just acute renal failure anymore? *Crit Care Nurse.* 2011;31(1):37–50.

Dirkes S. M. Continuous renal replacement therapy: dialysis for critically ill patients. *Am Nurse Today.* 2014;9(5):8–11.

Golestaneh L, Richter B, Amato-Hayes M. Logistics of renal replacement therapy: relevant issues for critical care nurses. *Am J Crit Care.* 2012;21(2):126–130.

Gomez NJ. Nephrology nursing process of care apheresis and therapeutic plasma exchange and continuous renal replacement therapy. Pitman, NJ: American Association of Nephrology Nurses' Association; 2011:21–39.

Graham P, Lischer E. Nursing issues in renal replacement therapy: organization, manpower assessment, competency evaluation and quality improvement processes. *Semin Dial.* 2011;24(2):183–187.

Maynar Moliner J, Honore PM, Sánchez-Izquierdo Riera JA, Herrera Gutiérrez M, Spapen HD. Handling continuous renal replacement therapy-related adverse effects in intensive care unit patients: the dialytrauma concept. *Blood Purif.* 2012;34(2):177–185.

Mottes T, Owens T, Niedner M, Juno J, Shanley TP, Heung M. Improving delivery of continuous renal replacement therapy: impact of a simulation-based educational intervention. *Pediatr Crit Care Med.* 2013;14(8):747–754.

Wiegand D, ed. *AACN Procedure Manual for Critical Care.* 6th ed. St Louis, MO: Elsevier Saunders; 2011:1018–1032.

Glossary

Access failure: it refers to obstruction within the catheter such that blood aspiration and/or flush is not adequate for RRT to function.

Blood in-flow pressure sensor (upstream blood pump-even known as access pressure sensor): it monitors the negative pressure between the patient's vascular access and the blood pump.

Activated partial thromboplastin time (APTT): a laboratory test used to monitor the degree of anticoagulation achieved with heparin.

Acute liver failure: is a syndrome in which rapid loss of metabolic and synthetic liver function leads to the hepatic encephalopathy and multi-organ failure in patients with no previous history of liver disease.

Acute on chronic liver failure: is a syndrome that occurs in patients with long-standing liver failure and cirrhosis of the liver where there is an acute decompensation of their disease process.

Adsorption: this term refers to the removal of molecules from the circulation independent of diffusion or convection, by binding of the molecules to the spongy layer of the filtering membrane.

Adverse event: an unexpected and undesirable outcome caused by the CRRT procedure. It may include premature filter clotting and obstruction with blood loss, patient bleeding due to excessive anticoagulation, hypovolaemia due to incorrect fluid balance settings, arrhythmia due to inappropriate electrolyte or volume management, hypotension due to incorrect fluid management, induction of electrolyte or acid base disorders due to incorrect fluid composition, or other similar unwanted complications of CRRT.

Air removal chamber (or air trap or bubble trap): a component of the CRRT circuit, located after the filter, to prevent air entry into the circuit, which would risk embolizing into the extracorporeal circuit or the patient's circulation.

Air-blood interface: a pocket of gas above the level of blood in the air removal chamber. This interface exposes blood to this gas and promotes clotting. The gas is initially air at the start of RRT, and enriches with carbon dioxide when bicarbonate fluids are used as substitution solution and heat liberates carbon dioxide.

Albumin dialysis: a form of artificial liver support where serum albumin is used as a component of the dialysate to enhance protein-bound toxin removal.

Anticoagulant/specific antagonist pumps: infuse anticoagulants/specific antagonists into the blood circuit. Based on the anticoagulation therapy, they can be further divided in systemic anticoagulation pumps (e.g. heparin), regional anticoagulation pumps (e.g. citrate) and reversal anticoagulation pumps (e.g. calcium). If necessary, specific antagonist drugs can be infused via a separate pump into the blood out-flow line (i.e., protamine).

Anticoagulant: a term used to describe any agent given to decrease blood clotting.

Artificial liver support: any device designed to specifically purify liver-related toxins, which may be responsible for the metabolic encephalopathy and multi-organ failure induced by liver failure.

Assessment of fluid status: this term refers to the clinical process of estimating the patient's intra- and extra-vascular fluid volume. Such assessment is complex and imperfect. It requires review of previous and current fluid balance and weight; consideration of vital signs; assessment of capillary refill and presence or absence of warm extremities; assessment of central venous pressure or neck veins; invasive and non-invasive, static or dynamic hemodynamic measurements; information on the effects of fluid therapy; radiological information; urinary output monitoring; measurement of blood lactate levels; and assessment of their changes over time and in response to therapy. Such assessment is necessary to guide fluid balance prescription during CRRT. Because of its complexity, such assessment is typically the source of much debate and disagreement at the bedside. The overriding principle of ICU fluid management is to ensure adequate tissue perfusion and to prevent intra- and extra-vascular fluid overload or depletion.

Backfiltration: it describes the movement of fluid from the dialysate compartment to the blood compartment due to local "negative" TMP (when pressure in dialysate/ ultrafiltrate compartment is higher than blood compartment pressure). Backfiltration usually is localized along the distal part of the filter.

Bioartificial liver support: any form of liver support which use filters impregnated with human or animal (usually porcine) liver cells (hepatocytes) to perform the three main functions of the liver: detoxification, biosynthesis and regulation.

Blood circulating phase: before starting the *treatment* phase, blood is circulated into the extracorporeal circuit (in this stage, the blood pump works but other pumps don't). An operator checklist is required to evaluate treatment parameters, appropriate air removal chamber blood level, and to avoid circuit bubbles.

Blood flow rate (Q_B): it is the volume of blood circulating into the extracorporeal circuit per unit of time, expressed in milliliters per minute (ml/min). During a treatment the configurable blood flow depends on the modality used, the type and quality of the vascular access and the hemodynamic stability of the patient.

Blood flow reduction: it identifies a blood flow less than set or prescribed, due to access catheter outflow failure and insufficient stroke volume of the roller pump tubing. It is usually associated with increasing negative blood in-flow pressure. Often, operator may remain unaware as pump rotation may remain stable.

Blood Leakage Detector (BLD): placed on the effluent line, monitors unwanted blood leaks from the blood compartment of the filter. Leak is caused by membrane rupture.

Blood pump: it is the pump that drives the blood through the extracorporeal circuit.

Blood purification: this term refers to the use of extracorporeal therapies such as CRRT for the treatment of a variety of conditions (drug overdose, liver failure, volume overload, diuretic resistant cardiac failure, severe sepsis) where a biological rationale exists for their application.

Blood return phase: this procedure is performed to return the blood to the patient. This is usually performed by connecting a saline solution bag to the blood in-flow line and running the blood pump.

Bolus dose: drug administration aimed at achieving therapeutic blood levels quickly. A continuous infusion at a lower dose is then provided to maintain this level.

Bubble detector: transducer that detects the presence of air in the blood out-flow line.

Catheter tip culture: assessment of a catheter tip (e.g. access catheter) for microbiological culture to identify the presence of catheter colonization.

Circuit life: an equivalent term for filter life. It is probably a more correct term than *filter life* because some circuits develop obstruction to adequate blood flow because of clot, clogging or both, elsewhere in the circuit and not in the filter itself.

Citrate: a molecule administered to chelate (bind) calcium in the extracorporeal circuit blood and make it unavailable as a co-factor in the activation of the clotting process. The majority of infused citrate is dialyzed or ultrafiltered out of the system, with bound calcium. Remaining citrate enters the patient, where the liver and muscle metabolize it into bicarbonate. The calcium lost into the effluent or ultrafiltrate (bound to citrate) is then replaced by a separate infusion of calcium. Citrate acts as both an anticoagulant and a buffer when it converts into bicarbonate. The amount given is sufficient to inhibit clotting within the circuit but typically does not have an effect on systemic anticoagulation.

Connection to the patient: this phase consists of the connection of the extracorporeal lines to the patient vascular access. The procedure must be performed keeping aseptic conditions.

Continuous Veno-Venous Hemodiafiltration (CVVHDF): this therapy combines hemodialysis and hemofiltration modalities.

Continuous Veno-Venous Hemodialysis (CVVHD): a modality of continuous HD characterized by slow counter-current/co-current dialysate flow into the dialysate compartment of the hemodialyzer. The main mechanism of transmembrane solute transport is diffusion.

Continuous Veno-Venous Hemofiltration (CVVH): a modality of continuous HF. The mechanism of transmembrane solute transport is convection.

Continuous Veno-Venous high-flux Hemodialysis (CVVHFD): it consists of the same modality as in CVVHD but carried out utilizing high-flux membranes. Due to the high-flux properties of the membrane, a convective component of solute clearance is achieved even if replacement fluid is not infused.

Convection: it is the process whereby solutes pass through the membrane's pores dragged by fluid movement (ultrafiltration); fluid movement is driven by a hydrostatic or osmotic transmembrane pressure gradient.

Cut-Off: for a specific membrane, the cut-off point represents the range of molecular weights of the smallest solutes retained by the membranes. Taking into account the normal distribution of membranes' pore size, the statistical cut-off value is identified as the molecular weight of the solute with a sieving coefficient of 0.1. It mainly depends on pore dimensions and geometry.

Delivered Dose: the delivered dose or real dose is the clinically relevant amount of (measured) clearance delivered to the patient. It mainly depends on specific RRT modality, treatment settings and other technical and clinical issues that qualitatively and quantitatively affect clearance, including: differences between the displayed and real flows of blood or effluent rate; adequacy of vascular access; adequacy of priming procedure; potential loss of surface area (by clotting or air); adsorption to the membrane; loss of permeability (clotting of the membrane, protein cake deposition on the inner surface of membranes, concentration polarization); high blood viscosity and hematocrit; and excessive filtration fraction.

Dialysate pump: it is the pump that drives the dialysate into the hemodialyzer.

Dialysate flow rate (Q_D): it is the amount of dialysis fluid running into the circuit per unit of time (minutes, hours). Q_D is measured in ml/h.

Dialysate volume(V_D) it is the amount of dialysis fluid running into the hemodialyzer during the whole treatment. V_D is expressed in milliliters (ml).

Dialysis: the separation of substances across a semipermeable membrane on the basis of particle size and concentration gradients.

Diffusion: it is a process whereby molecules move across a membrane in all directions. Statistically, this movement results in the passage of solutes from a more concentrated to a less concentrated area until equilibrium concentration between the two sites is reached. The concentration gradient ($C_1 - C_2 = dc$) is the driving force.

Direct (or internal) filtration: direct filtration identifies the one-directional movement of plasma water from the blood-side to the dialysate/ultrafiltrate side of the filter due to local positive TMP (I): plasma water is removed from blood and transferred into the dialysate compartment. Direct filtration takes place in the proximal section of the filter, until a critical point along the length of the filter is reached, when TMP (I)=0.

Disconnection phase: in a CRRT treatment, procedure of disconnection of the tubes from the vascular access of the patient.

Disposables (consumables): components that together make a functioning system and, in the case of CRRT, a circuit. Commonly, disposable plastic pieces connecting together are known as disposables or consumables.

Diuretic resistance: this term refers to conditions where marked edema (anasarca) develops despite intensive, high dose, multiple diuretic-based attempts to remove excess fluid.

Downtime: it is the time when the CRRT machine treatment is stopped. Interruptions during the treatment can occur due to machine alarms, circuit clotting, vascular access malfunctions or when patient requires procedures performed outside the intensive care unit, i.e. surgery or radiological investigations.

Dry weight: this is the patient's normal/optimal weight before the onset of illness. This weight is often available in detail in elective operative patients where it is typically measured before the operation. In other cases, it might need to be estimated.

Edema: this term refers to the accumulation of excess fluid in the extracellular compartment. In the subcutaneous tissue, it can be detected by the phenomenon of pitting of the skin under pressure. In the lungs, if significant, it can be detected by radiography. CT scanning may detect brain or intestinal edema. Edema of other organs (heart, liver, kidney) is likely important but cannot be detected unless extreme.

Effective time of treatment: it is the cumulative time while the effluent pump is working.

Efficacy: measures the effective removal of a specific solute resulting from a given treatment in a given patient. It can be identified as the ratio of the entire volume cleared during the treatment to the volume of distribution of that solute. Operatively, efficacy is a dimensionless number that it can be numerically defined as the ratio between intensity and the volume of distribution of a specific solute.

Efficiency: identified as a clearance (K), the efficiency represents the volume of blood cleared of a solute over a given period of time. It can be expressed as the ratio of blood volume over time (ml/min, ml/h, l/h, l/24h, etc.) and is generally normalized to ideal patient weight (ml/Kg/h).

Effluent flow rate (QEFF): it is the effluent volume coming from the exit (outflow) port on side of the filter per unit of time (minutes, hours). It is expressed in ml/h. Quantitatively it can be expressed as:

$$Q_{EFF} = Q_{UF} + Q_D = Q_{UF}^{NET} + Q_R + Q_D$$

Effluent volume (V_{EFF}): measured in ml/h, it represents the waste fluids coming from the filter exit (outflow) port on the side of the filter. Quantitatively it can be expressed as:

$$V_{EFF} = V_{UF} + V_D = V_{UF}^{NET} + V_R + V_D$$

Effluent/ultrafiltrate pressure sensor: monitors the pressure in the effluent/ultrafiltrate side of the filter. It is placed before the effluent pump and allows calculating trans-membrane pressure.

Effluent/ultrafiltrate pump: is the pump that drives the removal of fluid from the filter.

Extracorporeal circuit (E.C.): the path for blood flow outside the body. Includes the plastic tubing carrying the blood to the filter from the access catheter and from the filter back to the body via the access catheter.

Filter: it is the key disposable where blood is effectively depurated. Historically, the designation *filter* describes the entire depurative extracorporeal device system (i.e. membranes, housing, etc.) and includes all the particular terms like hemofilter, hemo-dialyzer, hemodiafilter and plasmafilter.

Filter holder: holds the filter or the entire filter-tubing kit on the machine.

Filter life: it is defined as the time elapsed (h, min) between the start of blood flow through the filter and the time when blood is unable to pass through the filter due to clot formation and obstruction of the filter.

Filtration fraction (FF): it is defined as

$$FF = \frac{1 - Prot_{IN}}{Prot_{OUT}}$$

where $Prot_{IN}$ is the protein concentration in plasma entering the filter, while $Prot_{OUT}$ is the protein concentration in plasma exiting the filter. Anyway, a directly measurable value of FF can be estimated as the ratio between the ultrafiltration rate and the plasma flow rate expressed as a fraction:

$$FF = \frac{Q_{UF}}{Q_P} = \frac{Q_{UF}}{Q_B(1 - HCT) + Q_R^{PRE}}$$

where Q_R^{PRE} is the pre infusion rate. For practical clinical purposes, however, it is usually defined as the ratio of the ultrafiltration rate over the blood flow rate:

$$FF = \frac{Q_{UF}}{Q_B + Q_R^{PRE}}$$

Fluid control system: allows a direct monitoring of the treatment fluid balance. It can be gravimetric, volumetric, flowmetric or a combination of those mechanisms.

Free drug concentration: this term refers to the percentage or amount of a given drug that is not protein-bound. This concept is important because, in case of drug overdose with a water-soluble drug (e.g. lithium, virtually 0% protein bound, or sodium valpro-ate, 90-95% protein bound), only the free (unbound) drug is available for removal by CRRT.

Heater: heats the dialysate/replacement fluids, or the blood flowing through the blood out-flow line of the extracorporeal circuit.

Hemodiafilter (or diafilter): filter designed for hemodiafiltration modality.

Hemodiafiltration (HDF): combines both HD and HF, whereby the mechanisms involved in solute removal are both diffusive and convective.

Hemodialysis (HD): the main mechanism of solute removal in hemodialysis is diffusion, which is especially effective in the removal of small solutes. HD involves the use of a hemodialyzer where blood and an appropriate dialysate solution circulate counter-current or co-current to each other.

Hemodialyzer (or dialyzer): filter designed for hemodialysis modality.

Hemofilter: filter designed for hemofiltration modality.

Hemofiltration (HF): it is an exclusively ultrafiltration/convection treatment, where no dialysis fluid is used. Infusion of a sterile solution into the blood circuit replaces the reduced plasma volume and reduces solute concentration. Infusion of a sterile solution (replacement fluid) can replace totally or partially the filtered volume. Replacement fluid can be infused pre-filter (Pre-Dilution) or post-filter (Post-Dilution).

Hemoperfusion (HP): in hemoperfusion, blood circulates through a column containing specific sorbents; adsorption is the only removal mechanism.

Heparin coating: administering the drug heparin into the circuit priming solution with the aim of preventing clotting due to blood contact with plastic surfaces where the heparin has coated the surface.

Heparin: a drug commonly used to prevent blood clotting within the extracorporeal circuit.

High-cut off hemofiltration: this modality refers to the use of high-cut off membranes in hemofilters to increase CRRT's ability to remove soluble mediators in patients with sepsis. This therapy is controversial; no trials have shown evidence of clinical benefit.

High-cut off membranes: this term describes membranes with a cut-off value that approximates the molecular weight of albumin.

High-flux hemodialysis (HFD): it is a HD with high flux membranes and it can achieve significant ultrafiltration/convective transport.

High flux membranes: membranes with a $K_{UF} > 25$ml/h/mmHg/m^2

High-volume hemofiltration: this term refers to a CRRT modality where the convective delivered dose is higher than 35 ml/Kg/h. The goal of such therapy is to increase the intensity of blood purification to address not just renal dysfunction, but also humoral components of sepsis (cytokines) whose removal from the circulation may be desirable. This therapy is controversial; recent trials have shown lack of clinical benefit.

Humoral theory of sepsis: this term refers to a particular framework of biological thinking used to explain the clinical manifestations of severe sepsis. According to this theory, the severe sepsis or septic shock syndrome is due to an excessive release of cytokines into the blood stream. This conceptual framework provides the rationale for using CRRT in sepsis.

International normalized ratio for the prothrombin time(INR): this test is used to measure and monitor the degree of anticoagulation achieved with warfarin. It is frequently prolonged in patients with liver disease and may be used to guide the (sometimes unnecessary) need for additional anticoagulant treatment in such patients.

Intensity: it can be defined by the product "Efficiency X Time". Operatively, intensity represents the blood volume cleared of a solute after a certain period of time; it can be expressed as ml or l.

Isolated Ultrafiltration (iUF): the main goal of iUF is to remove fluid by ultrafiltration, utilizing highly permeable membranes without volume replacement. Isolated ultrafiltration removes solutes in terms of mass, rather than concentration (solvent drag).

Light and buzzer indicators: visual and auditory alarms must be clear and comprehensive. The different priorities of the alarms should be univocally categorized according to a specific standard.

Liver support devices: any artificial device to purify blood in the setting of liver failure. This term encompasses both artificial and bioartificial liver support systems.

Low flux membranes: membranes with a $K_{UF} < 10ml/h/mmHg/m^2$

Low molecular weight heparin (LMWH): a drug that is a modification of the naturally occurring unfractionated heparin molecule, which can be used to achieve circuit anticoagulation during CRRT. It can be given as a single subcutaneous dose once a day. Various types of LMWH exist and some can accumulate in patients with kidney failure, thus its activity should be monitored daily by assays for anti-factor Xa activity rather than the aPTT. The effects of LMWH can only be partially reversed by protamine.

Machine (CRRT) fluid balance: this term refers to the total balance over a 24 hour period of fluids infused into the CRRT circuit (dialysate, replacement fluid or both, depending on the technique and (any) additional anticoagulant infusion) and fluids removed by the CRRT machine into the effluent (ultrafiltration).

Mass transfer area coefficient (K_0A): it represents the overall capacity of the membrane to remove a solute by diffusion over the entire filter surface. It is defined as the product of the solute flux per unit of membrane area (K_0) and the entire membrane surface area. The unit of measure is ml/min.

Membrane porosity(ρ): it is function of number and size of pores. It can be approximated as $\rho = N_p \cdot \pi \cdot r_p^{-2}$, where N_p is the number of pores and r_p^- is mean pore radius. The mass transfer coefficient can be considered the intrinsic clearance of a filter-solute pair where clearance is the rate of solute removal per unit of gradient of solute concentration.

Middle flux membranes: membranes with a $10\ ml/h/mmHg/m^2 < K_{UF} < 25\ ml/h/mmHg/m^2$

Middle-molecular weight molecules: this term refers to all molecules that are > 0.5 kDa in molecular weight but less than albumin (66 kDa) in size. These molecules, if water-soluble, can theoretically, be removed by CRRT. Because of their size, they are more efficiently removed by convection than by diffusion. Many of these molecules are soluble mediators/cytokines.

Net ultrafiltration flow rate (Q_{UF}^{NET}): it is the net amount of fluid extracted from the patient per unit of time·Q_{UF}^{NET} is expressed in liters per hour (ml/h) or grams per hour (g/h)·Q_{UF}^{NET} can also be expressed as Δ *weight rate* or *weight loss rate* when referred to the treatment and not to the patient.

Net ultrafiltration volume(V_{UF}^{NET}): it is the net amount of fluid withdrawn/removed from the patient, measured in milliliters (ml)·V_{UF}^{NET} can be expressed as ml or grams (g) since the density of plasma water can be approximated to 1 Kg/dm³ (1 g = 1 ml)· V_{UF}^{NET} can also be expressed as Δ *weight* or *weight loss* when referred to the treatment and not to the patient.

No anticoagulation: in patients considered at high risk of bleeding because of recent major surgery, low platelet count, abnormal clotting tests or any combination of these can receive CRRT without the administration of any anticoagulant drug.

Orgaran: this drug is a low molecular weight glycosaminoglycan, which can be used to anticoagulate the circuit in the presence of the heparin induced thrombocytopenia thrombosis syndrome (HITTS).

Patient fluid balance: this term refers to the total balance over a 24-hour period of fluids administered (intermittent drugs, continuous infusions of drugs, blood, blood products, nutrient solutions, additional fluids) minus measurable fluids removed (drainage from chest or abdomen, urine – if present, blood loss and excess fluid removed by the CRRT machine).

Plasma flow rate (Q_P): it is the volume of plasma circulating into the extracorporeal circuit per unit of time, expressed in milliliters per minute (ml/min). It can be approximated as:

$$Q_P = (1 - HCT) Q_B$$

where *HCT* is hematocrit and Q_B the blood flow.

Post dialysate pump pressure sensor: monitors the pressure in the dialysate line before the connection with the filter. It permits a better estimate of transmembrane pressure.

Post Infusion (Q_R^{POST}): in post infusion (or post dilution or post-filter infusion) modalities, replacement fluid is infused downstream the filter.

Pre filter pressure sensor (downstream blood pump): located between blood pump and filter, it monitors the positive blood pressure and allows calculating transmembrane pressure and pressure drop in the filter.

Pre Infusion (Q_R^{PRE}): in pre infusion (or pre dilution or pre-filter infusion) modalities, the replacement fluid is infused upstream of the filter.

Preparation phase: it includes the collection of the necessary disposable material, the identification and control of the disposable set, set charge (cassette tubing), connection to the filter, positioning of tubing, and hanging of bags and tubes connection.

Pre-Post Infusion ($Q_R^{PRE/POST}$): in pre-post infusion (or pre-post dilution or pre-post filter infusion) modalities, replacement fluid is infused both upstream and downstream the filter. The ratio of the upstream to downstream infusion can be modulated to achieve the optimal compromise to maximize clearance while avoiding the consequences of a high TMP and hemoconcentration.

Pre replacement pump pressure sensor: monitors the negative pressure before the replacement pump. It provides information about the ability of the pump to obtain fluids from its bags.

Prescription phase: during CRRT, it includes decisions on required modality and related operational parameters. It includes even a periodic reassessment and/or change of the prescription.

Priming phase: priming solution is infused into extracorporeal circuit in order to remove air. When heparin anticoagulation is used, it is usually added into the priming solution. During this phase, the machine makes a general check of all components and sensors.

Priming volume of the filter (V_b): **represents the volume of the blood compartment of the filter. It can be approximated as** $V_b = N_f \cdot L \cdot \pi \cdot r_i^{\sigma 2}$ **, where** N_f is the number of fibers, L the length of fibers and r_i^σ the mean inner radius of the fibers.

Prostacyclin: a drug that interferes with platelet aggregation and can be used as a continuous infusion to retard circuit clotting during CRRT.

Protamine: a drug given to bind heparin and to reverse its anticoagulant effect. The typical effective ratio for full heparin effect blockade is 1 mg of protamine for each 100 international units of heparin. Protamine can be given to reverse the effect of heparin within the circuit, before blood is returned to the patient.

Regional anticoagulation: any anticoagulation of the circuit but not of the patient. This might include the use of citrate with separate administration of calcium, or the use of heparin with simultaneous administration of protamine post-filter, to reverse its effect before the blood is returned to the patient.Rejection Coefficient (*RC*): it is defined as:

$$RC = 1 - SC$$

where SC is the sieving coefficient

Replacement flow rate(Q_R): it is the amount of fluid replaced into the CRRT circuit per time interval (minute, hour). Q_R is usually measured in ml/h.

Replacement/infusion pump: is the pump that drives the flow of replacement fluid into the blood in-flow line (predilution, usually between the blood pump and the filter) and/or into the blood out-flow line (postdilution, usually in the air removal chamber).

Replacement volume(V_R): it is the amount of fluid (milliliters) replaced either upstream (pre infusion or pre dilution) or downstream (post infusion or post dilution) or both (pre-post infusion or pre-post dilution) of the filter into the RRT circuit.

Air removal chamber clotting: clot formation in the circuit air removal chamber, sited between the filter and the patient's vascular access.

Safety electroclamp: produces a safety occlusion in blood out-flow line when air is detected by the bubble detector.

Screen: the monitor through which the user interacts with the machine (ensuring good visualization and good maneuverability). Software operator interface must allow a complete, easy and friendly access to all the required information.

Sieving coefficient (SC): it is the ratio of a specific solute concentration in the ultrafiltrate (removed solely by convective mechanism) over the mean solute concentration in the plasma before and after the filter:

$$SC = 2 \cdot \frac{C_{UF}}{C_{P_i} + C_{P_o}}$$

SC is specific for each solute and for every specific membrane. It is common to simplify this formula into the ratio between the concentration in the ultrafiltrate and the solute concentration in the plasma before the filter.

Slow Continuous Ultra Filtration (SCUF): it is a therapy based only on slow removal of plasma water based on ultrafiltration.

Snap shot data: data collected to measure clinical care or outcomes during a short period of time, designed to provide a quick picture that might suggest a longer-term behavior, trend or outcome.

Soluble mediators: this term refers to molecules (mostly small to medium-sized peptides), which participate in the pathogenesis of the pro- and anti-inflammatory responses seen after major body injury or infection. These molecules are water soluble and therefore potentially removable by CRRT. Many of these molecules are called "cytokines".

Sorbent: even called cartridge or adsorber, this device doesn't belong to the category of filters and adsorption is the only purifying modality.

Special procedures: during treatment, special procedures include replenishment of dialysate, replacement fluid, regional anticoagulation bags (e.g. when citrate anticoagulation is used) and exchange of syringes (e.g. when using heparin anticoagulation), temporary disconnection, recirculation, and replacement of filter and kit

Surface area of a filter (A): **represents the total area of membrane directly in contact with blood. It can be approximated as** $A = 2 \cdot N_f \cdot L \cdot \pi \cdot r_i^\sigma$ **, where** N_f is the number of fibers, L the length of fibers and r_i^σ the mean inner radius of the fibers.

Systemic anticoagulation: where an administered anticoagulant has a direct effect on the patient's ability to activate the clotting cascade. The delay of the coagulation is monitored by blood tests specific for the agent used.

Target Prescribed dose: it is the amount of clearance the physician desires to set in the machine. It is the only value that can be set in the machine. The target delivered dose is usually set as a target delivered efficiency or by specifying the flow settings and RRT modality.

Total time of treatment: it is defined as the sum of the effective time of treatment and downtime.

Transmembrane pressure (TMP): in hollow fibers filters, TMP is the pressure gradient across the membranes. The terms that define TMP are the hydrostatic pressure (P_B) in the blood compartment, the hydrostatic pressure (P_D) in the dialysate-ultrafiltrate compartment and the oncotic pressure (π_B). Generally, *TMP* is expressed using a simplified formula:

$$TMP^* = \frac{P_{Bi} + P_{Bo}}{2} - \frac{P_{Di} + P_{Do}}{2} - \frac{\pi_{Bi} + \pi_{Bo}}{2}$$

where P_{Bi} is blood inlet pressure, P_{Bo} is blood outlet pressure, P_{Di} is dialysate/ultrafiltrate inlet pressure, P_{Do} is dialysate/ultrafiltrate outlet pressure, π_{Bi} is oncotic pressure of blood inlet, π_{Bo} is oncotic pressure of blood outlet.

Furthermore, usually the CRRT machines don't have a direct measurement of the dialysate inlet pressure (P_{Di}) and can't measure the oncotic pressure; so the TMP is calculated through a further simpler formula:

$$TMP^{**} = \frac{P_{Bi} + P_{Bo}}{2} - P_{EFF}$$

where P_{EEF} is the pressure measured in the effluent line by the machine.

Treatment phase: it is the phase where blood purification is properly performed and ultrafiltration and diffusive and/or convective solute transport are activated (all the pumps work). Patient vital signs and circuit pressures must be monitored throughout the treatment phase.

Ultrafiltrate volume (V_{UF}: measured in milliliters (ml), it is the total amount of fluid removed by positive TMP in the filter during a RRT treatment. V_{UF} depends on various extracorporeal circuit parameters, including blood flow, filter and fiber design, TMP, membrane ultrafiltration coefficient and surface area. V_R and V_{UF}^{NET}, determine the ultrafiltrate volume V_{UF}:

$$V_{UF} = V_R + V_{UF}^{NET}$$

Ultrafiltration: is the phenomenon of transport of plasma water (solvent) through a semi-permeable membrane, driven by a hydraulic pressure gradient between blood and dialysate compartments.

Ultrafiltration coefficient of the membrane (KUF): represents the water permeability of filter's membranes per unit of pressure and surface. It depends on the dimension and the number of the pores. The unit of measure is ml/h/mmHg/m². Therefore, treatment parameters, which enhance or reduce pore blockage will induce change in the value of K_{UF}. K_{UF} is empirically and practically measured as:

$$K_{UF} = \frac{Q_{UF}}{TMP} \cdot \frac{1}{A}$$

where Q_{UF} is the ultrafiltration flow rate, TMP is transmembrane pressure and A is the membranes surface area.

Ultrafiltration Coefficient of the filter (DKUF): it is defined as the product of the ultrafiltration coefficient of the membrane K_{UF} times membranes surface area (A):

$$DK_{UF} = K_{UF} \cdot A$$

The unit of measure is ml/h/mmHg.

DK_{UF} can be empirically and practically measured by membrane manufacturers as the ratio between the ultrafiltration rate (Q_{UF}) obtained and the applied transmembrane pressure TMP.

Ultrafiltration flow rate (Q_{UF}): it is the amount of ultrafiltrate produced per time interval (minute, hour). The unit of measure is milliliters per hour (ml/h). Q_{UF} is prescribed to achieve a desired V_{UF} within the scheduled treatment duration (usually 24 hours).

Unload phase: in a CRRT treatment, procedure of unloading of the disposables from the hardware of the machine.

Index

Tables, figures and boxes are indicated by an italicized *t*, *f* or *b*, respectively.

303